"I found so many resonances with my own experiences in Suzanne Braun Levine's book. And the information is astonishing. *Inventing the Rest of Our Lives* will have a huge impact and will clarify so many things for so many women."

—Carol Gilligan, Ph.D., author of *In a Different Voice* and *The Birth of Pleasure*

"Like a series of rare, deeply insightful, and deeply meaningful conversations with very wise friends, *Inventing the Rest of Our Lives* gives us an entirely new perspective on our own lives as we reshape what it means to be fifty and beyond."

—Ellen Galinsky, President, Families and Work Institute

"If you are fifty, sixty, seventy, or older or if you plan to reach those ages, this is the book for you. Levine does not ignore the brambles on the path of life, even as she encourages us to pluck the flowers. Practical, unsentimental, and inspiring, this book illuminates the way forward."

—Carol Tavris, Ph.D., author of *The Mismeasure of Woman*

Inventing the Rest of Our Lives

ALSO BY SUZANNE BRAUN LEVINE

Father Courage: What Happens When Men Put Family First

Inventing the Rest of Our Lives

WOMEN IN SECOND ADULTHOOD

Suzanne Braun Levine

VIKING

VIKING
Published by the Penguin Group
Penguin Group (USA) Inc., 375 Hudson Street, New York, New York 10014, U.S.A. · Penguin
Group (Canada), 10 Alcorn Avenue, Toronto, Ontario, Canada M4V 3B2 · (a division of Pearson
Penguin Canada Inc.) · Penguin Books Ltd, 80 Strand, London WC2R 0RL, England · Pen-
guin Ireland, 25 St. Stephen's Green, Dublin 2, Ireland (a division of Penguin Books Ltd) ·
Penguin Books Australia Ltd, 250 Camberwell Road, Camberwell, Victoria 3124, Australia (a di-
vision of Pearson Australia Group Pty Ltd) · Penguin Books India Pvt Ltd, 11 Community Cen-
tre, Panchsheel Park, New Delhi–110 017, India · Penguin Group (NZ), Cnr Airborne and
Rosedale Roads, Albany, Auckland 1310, New Zealand (a division of Pearson New Zealand
Ltd) · Penguin Books (South Africa) (Pty) Ltd, 24 Sturdee Avenue, Rosebank, Johannesburg
2196, South Africa

Penguin Books Ltd, Registered Offices: 80 Strand, London WC2R 0RL, England

First published in 2005 by Viking Penguin, a member of Penguin Group (USA) Inc.

10 9 8 7 6 5 4 3 2 1

Grateful acknowledgment is made for permission to reprint excerpts from the following copy-
righted works:
    "Weathering" from *Poems 1960–2000* by Fleur Adcock (Bloodaxe Books, 2000). By permis-
sion of the author.
    "Leap Before You Look" from *Collected Poems* by W. H. Auden. Copyright 1945 by W. H.
Auden. Used by permission of Random House, Inc.
    "Falling in Love at 55" by Ellen Bass. © Ellen Bass, 2004. By permission of the author.
    "The Journey" from *Dream Work* by Mary Oliver. Copyright © 1986 by Mary Oliver. Used
by permission of Grove/Atlantic, Inc.

LIBRARY OF CONGRESS CATALOGING IN PUBLICATION DATA
Levine, Suzanne.
    Inventing the rest of our lives : women in second adulthood / Suzanne Braun Levine.
        p.   cm.
    Includes bibliographical references and index.
    ISBN 0-670-03311-1
    1. Middle-aged women—Psychology.   2. Older women—Psychology.   3. Self-
actualization (Psychology).   I. Title.
    HQ1059.4.L48 2005
    05.244'2—dc22   2004049623

This book is printed on acid-free paper. ∞

Printed in the United States of America

For my mother,

ESTHER BERNSON BRAUN

Acknowledgments

After more than thirty-five years of marriage, there are few surprises, but my husband Bob Levine's editorial acumen has been a delightful one for me and an essential contribution to this book. The expert pushing and pulling from a brilliant editor, Janet Goldstein, and a devoted agent, Janis Donnaud, also challenged me to do better. I thank you all.

And to Steve and Cynthia Rubin who contributed an actual "room of one's own" to work in and to those others who kept the details under control—Karen Grenke, Rebecca Hart, Paula Marsili, and Rachel Rapkin—thank you too.

Most of all, I am grateful to the women who shared their stories and the friends in my "circle of trust" who provide all good things.

Contents

Moving On to What's Next:
Making Peace and Taking Charge

Getting to What Matters: Letting Go and Saying No

CHAPTER ONE

You're Not Who You Were, Only Older

The sense of danger must not disappear:
The way is certainly both short and steep,
However gradual it looks from here;
Look if you like, but you will have to leap.
. . .
Much can be said for savoir-faire,
But to rejoice when no one else is there
Is even harder than it is to weep;
No one is watching, but you have to leap.
. . .
Our dream of safety has to disappear.

—W. H. Auden, "Leap Before You Look"

My first step into Second Adulthood was backward off a ninety-foot cliff. On impulse, I had signed up for an Outward Bound program and found myself poised in full rappelling gear—harness, helmet, and guide rope—to walk down the face of what could just as well have been my twelve-story apartment building. The terror was pure. I was only mildly distracted by the reassuring words of our leader: "Fear is the appropriate response here. After all, evolution doesn't take much interest in creatures that step backward off ninety-foot cliffs."

I made it down, of course. I had learned the lesson the exercise was surely designed to teach, that fear is not an unacceptable response, but it can be confronted. And I fulfilled a personal mission: to find out if I was still a Tomboy. (The very word, I realize as I use it, is a throwback to a bygone era, not just my own past.) My tomboy self, long lost in a marriage to a nonathletic, non–nature-lover and a busy urban life, played a big part in my personal mythology. Ever since I crossed the fiftieth birthday barrier a couple of years earlier I had wanted to reconnect with that rugged, adventurous outdoorswoman, if indeed she was still an authentic component of who I am. If my tomboy *was* still there, I wanted to share that part of me with my daughter, who was growing up in a time more accepting of the "big-boned" body type we share and as a young woman with an unequivocal appreciation of her body's strength. But first I had to make sure I wasn't perpetuating a myth about myself. Having grown up feeling I was often playing a part written by others, I wanted, as best I could, to get to the truth about my life.

As my feet hit the ground and I looked back up the craggy cliff toward the blue sky and my cheering companions, I was overcome with emotion—emotions really, more than I can identify even now—and I began to sob and laugh uncontrollably. But it was after I calmed down and had gone kind of limp that a totally unexpected breakthrough of really cosmic proportions hit. The descent down the cliff came on the fifth day of a seven-day program. I had done everything asked of me—jumping into icy water at dawn, sleeping on oars lined across an open boat, climbing a telephone pole, swinging on a rope into a spider-web net—so I was primed to obediently take on the next assignment. It was to keep our harnesses and ropes in place and climb back *up* the wall. Maybe it was because I was so totally wasted by the emotional and physical exertion, but I would like to think it was overcoming fear on the way down that gave me the courage to say *no* to going back up.

The only others in the group who declined to climb were two women in their fifties. We realized with some astonishment that, for us, saying no was as monumental an achievement as stepping backward off the cliff. Both challenges were more meaningful to the three of us because we were women of a certain age. Each of us had a different reason for coming to the wilderness, yet we shared an awakening drive to sort out our thinking about the next stage of our lives. In our dealings with that cliff we had encountered two essential themes of Second Adulthood: *Letting Go* and *Saying No*.

Letting Go and Saying No

In my lexicon, Second Adulthood is the unprecedented and productive time that our generation is encountering as we pass that dreaded landmark of a fiftieth birthday. If you think of your first adulthood as, roughly, the twenty-five years in which you built your life and set your style, the next twenty-five years can be a second chance—to do it better, to do it differently, to do it wiser. I say *can be* because a lot depends on luck—good health, good fortune, good friends. But a lot also depends on determination—taking risks, making change, weighing new options.

To seize that second chance requires recalibrating many of the primary forces in our lives and shifting gears. As anyone in our age group knows, to shift gears you first have to disengage the clutch and literally give up control for a moment. In the context of the Second Adulthood transition, letting go—of worn-out demands, of old news, of empty promises—is like stepping backward off a cliff. It is terrifying, especially for women who have spent a lifetime holding on, keeping things together, planning, coordinating, and prioritizing. It is hard to surrender to serendipity and to risk and change. It is distressing to find oneself having to renegotiate the most intimate relationships. But whether we see it as an adventure or not, we are at an age when circumstances force us to let go—of our children, of our looks, of some of our life goals—and feel ourselves *fall apart,* to ease off doing what we know how to do, to look into the abyss. For those who take the leap, letting go is also an opportunity to consolidate, to cherish, and to soar out over new terrain.

Saying no is the assertive form of letting go. If letting go focuses on acceptance and release, saying no focuses on actively shedding baggage that is getting in the way of moving on. Eliminating what doesn't work for us anymore, talking back to people who have intimidated us in the past, renouncing behavior that doesn't feel authentic—all those noes are an important way of taking charge of our lives. They enable us to travel light toward clarity of purpose. Those first defiant noes are the prelude to many a triumphant yes! There's a catch, though—those triumphs can't be anticipated from the safety of solid ground. We have to take the plunge into Second Adulthood without knowing who we will be when we come up for air.

Reinventing Ourselves and Rewriting History

In many respects, we have been here before. Thirty years ago, at the beginning of our first adulthood, we were also on the verge of big changes; we were struggling to address what Betty Friedan had identified as *The Problem That Has No Name*—the dismissive and restrictive assumptions about women and their role in society. At that time, many women felt isolated and confused and guilty for not being satisfied with what they had been given, but fearful of talking about it.

Time and again, they found that the simple, yet risky, act of telling the truth about their doubts, failures, and fears to someone who appeared confident and accomplished resulted in a reassuring—and amazed—"me too!" response. In sharing frustration over household demands, impatience with children, anger at husbands, concerns about sexuality, and doubts about measuring up to media images, women found validation for their own perceptions, support, and the emotional high of not feeling like the only crazy woman on the block. One by one, those intimate revelations changed the conversation about women's roles as they changed each woman's own life.

The discovery that the personal is political—that our most private efforts have meaning in the community of women and impact beyond—led to the revolution that got us to this place. Today, motivated by that energy and those achievements, we are confronting a new unknown—The Problem That Has No Name has been replaced by The Question That Has Many Answers: *What am I going to do with the rest of my life?* Second Adulthood.

Second Adulthood is a *journey* each of us embarks on, but it is also a *stage* that our generation is in the process of defining as we live it. This book is about both. Sharing the stories of individual women's journeys gives reassurance to others; describing the parameters of the new life stage highlights the substantial upside of what can feel like a meltdown. There is great promise in Second Adulthood, but there is also an inescapable downside to getting older. A woman turning fifty this year has a 40 percent chance of living to one hundred, but she has the same chance of being erased from her world by Alzheimer's. Hormonal shifts can throw us off kilter into depression and anxiety, but they can also release a heady dose of defiance and energy, a second wind. Despite our professional breakthroughs, ageism is pervasive and insidious in our culture. Poverty among women increases with age. Some of this bad news we have to accept, but every day we encounter situations that can be turned around. As we zero in on what really matters in our lives *now*, we become better able to recognize—and make peace with—circumstances we cannot change and we become more experienced in taking charge of those we can and want to change.

My understanding of Second Adulthood is drawn from the insights of women with diverse life experiences—from the most traditional or ambitious to the most off-beat or spiritual, from celebrities to retirees—because I know that the baseline experience for each of us is more similar than different. In addition, it provides needed perspective to hear how others are coping with common problems in unfamiliar situations. I interviewed fifty women in depth and spoke with numerous others in that casual-yet-intimate kind of conversation women often strike up. I learned from every one. As Gloria Steinem has pointed out, "anyone who has experienced something is more expert in it than the experts."

I also sought out the professionals who are following our trajectory. They are finding patterns that illuminate our anecdotal accounts and set our experience in the larger context of social change. The broad message of my research is that both the personal and the societal status quo are being challenged. As we make our individual ripples, we are collectively creating a major paradigm shift that has consequences well beyond our own lives. Just as women did during the years of discovery and rebellion that began in the seventies—whether or not an individual considered herself a part of the Women's Movement—we are now rewriting history as we are reinventing ourselves.

The New Stage of Life

Almost thirty-seven million American women in our late forties, fifties, and sixties are the beneficiaries of scientific and health breakthroughs that are prolonging our active lives. At an average life expectancy of eighty-plus years, we are likely to live as adults almost as long again as we already have. This is a new era for women. The choices we have made so far have set the stage for this new era. The choices we each make will define it. Our numbers will call attention to it.

Born in the 1940s and 1950s, we were raised in a culture that had a limited view of women's prospects; then we spent our first adulthood breaking free of those narrow expectations. During the seventies and eighties, we became acquainted with what women could do, even if we didn't personally achieve all we could have. And many of us have achieved more than our mothers ever could have dreamed. As a result, we bring to our Second Adulthood a double awareness: a first adulthood full of experience in reinventing ourselves; and the conviction that women belong in the public sphere—the marketplace, the civic arena, the sports stadium—not only in the home.

Now the last frontier is before us—*the grandma assumption*. In our mothers' generation the conventional wisdom was that once a woman reached the change of life, her life stopped changing. What she had not done by fifty, she would never do. What she did afterward wouldn't matter to anyone but the grandchildren she would spoil rotten. We are already turning those assumptions around.

It's not that we aren't reveling in the joys of participating in a new life. "I feel like I have taken a lover," a doting grandmother confessed to me. "My heart flutters when my granddaughter calls. I daydream about her at work. I shop for the silliest gifts for her." It's just that the momentum of our event-ful, busy, productive first adulthoods is propelling us past an all-consuming granny role. "I'm a doctor, a teacher, a lover, a political activist, a friend—*and* a grandma," another woman protested. "But as much as I adore my grandchildren, they are not the defining part of my life."

We are mature achievers and late bloomers. We are taking on challenges and taking care of ourselves. Far from fading into the woodwork, we are full of surprises. Most of the women I talked to about the onset of Second Adulthood re-ported at least some of the surprises that I experienced on my Outward Bound adventure:

- an impulsive decision to do something out of character
- a willingness to take a calculated risk into the unknown
- a determination to make contact with one's authentic self and tap into the true passion there
- a desire to become a source of truth about women to the next generation
- the delicious freedom of looking the latest expectation—in a lifetime of expectations—in the eye and saying, "Not me. Not now!"

I don't think it is an accident that the triumphant tomboy I longed to reconnect with dates back to an earlier stage when I felt power and confidence and then lost it. Like just about every woman now over fifty, I experienced adolescence as a time of increasing self-doubt, of abandoned not-for-girls dreams and of limitations closing in. For girls today, and even for us, it is hard to conjure up the time when girls had to wear only skirts and play jump rope and learn to giggle and make every statement into a question—a time when they had to rein in the high spirits of grade school days and start concentrating on the serious business of learning to please other people.

When readers of *More* magazine, a publication for women over forty, were asked about their age, the majority said they felt their best years were ahead of them. What they liked about being older was "not worrying about what other people think" and "being more self-confident" and even "no more menstrual cycle." Their words sound like a celebration of the girlhood sense of power and independence that our generation had to renounce. Second Adulthood is, in part, about recapturing that earlier state of mind and—at last—growing with it. For women of our generation, this is a unique moment, a second chance at growing up strong.

When we gather for fiftieth and sixtieth birthdays, we ask each other if we are grown up yet. The answer is: Yes, we are grown up, but at the same time we are only halfway there. We are about to grow up again.

You Are Not Who You Were, Only Older

The most important discovery I've made about Second Adulthood is that a woman entering this new stage is not the same one who set up her first adulthood life. We are approaching the next frontier as women with new ideas and responses, whose priorities are changing. That's why answering the question *what's next?* is not as easy as it may appear. For example, despite all I had riding on that wilderness challenge, outdoor life is off my agenda. The tomboy trip has become irrelevant, as have many of the other long-standing items on my to-do (in life) list. It would be easy if what Gail Sheehy first identified (in *New Passages*) as Second Adulthood were really about the opportunity to do "everything you always wanted to do." But like me, many women find themselves staring blankly at their life lists and wondering why they are not enthusiastic about fulfilling those long-standing dreams. The truth is we have outgrown them. They are dreams of a past adulthood. "Everything you always wanted to do" has little bearing on what you are going to do next. Because you are simply not that *you* anymore. You are simply *not* who you once were, only older.

This can be terribly confusing. Allison, who considers herself a clear-thinking woman, found herself awash in mixed signals. After only a year at a job that should have felt like the crowning achievement of her career, she couldn't believe she was thinking about, of all things, retiring. Where had all her ambition gone? Why was she not able, as she put it, "to enjoy success"? Why did she suddenly want to be home for the high school years of her youngest child, when she had always maintained that the stimulation of work she loved made her a better mother? She felt she was losing her convictions as well as her drive. "I just want to stay home and paint and take courses," she said flatly, as if talking about someone she barely knew.

Other women described their own experiences of getting off track with equal bewilderment. Some could not explain new tastes in foods—or new sexual interests. Others found themselves "behaving badly" but not inclined to apologize. Several described behavior that ultimately opened up new prospects, but looked and felt inexplicable or flaky at the time. Sylvia, for example, comfortable in a midlevel executive job, was in the midst of sending out an e-mail to her friends and colleagues about an opening at the top of another organization when instead of pushing *send*, she picked up the phone and proposed herself (and got the job). And Sara, who fought like crazy during her divorce proceedings to keep her rambling apartment with the dark velvet furniture and towering book-shelves she loved, but the next thing she knew, she was longing for sunshine and cozy spaces. She now lives in a small suburban high-rise where she can grow geraniums in every window. Patricia, a nonpracticing Jew all her life, felt an inexplicable longing for "more mystery" in her religious life and, after much soul-searching and study, ultimately converted to Catholicism. Madeline retired in order to escape the city and spend more time making her garden grow, yet found herself drawn toward a different kind of gardening. She now teaches English as a Second Language in an inner city homeless shelter.

As the journey goes forward, this unfamiliar persona, this mischievous Tinkerbell at our ear, matures into the voice we count on most. It gets stronger, more authoritative, more philosophical, more courageous. "Old women are different from everyone else," wrote novelist Ursula LeGuin. "They tell the truth."

You Are Not Who You Were. Literally.

The reconstructed *you* is not a figment of your imagination. The dynamic that many women are reporting—new outlook, new confidence, new dreams—is supported by scientific research from many disciplines. What we are learning about our bodies tells us that nature has by no means abandoned us at this stage, and what is becoming understood about our style of behavior tells us we are not programmed to fade away. On the contrary, we might be as well or better suited to new challenges at this stage of life than before.

Some of the most spectacular news I will report comes from neurology labs where researchers are concluding that, contrary to conventional thinking, the aging brain is not just degenerating. In fact, it is generating in ways that are supportive of big achievements after midlife. Until very recently, it was thought that brain growth stops even before physical maturity and, in middle age, the brain begins a decline into a series of senior moments. While it is true that certain kinds of memory processes get rusty (I have a friend who claims that "these days, remembering a name is better than having an orgasm"), other capabilities begin gearing up at around age forty-five and continue for a decade or more. Specifically, in that part of the brain responsible for making judgments, finding new solutions to old problems, and managing emotions—not sweating the small stuff—there is a great leap forward.

I will also describe how medical science is only just beginning to address the ways that women's bodies get sick or stay well. Until now most of what we knew about heart attacks, for example, was based on the male model. It is now clear that heart attacks in women have been going undiagnosed because we present different symptoms. Our bodies age and adapt in ways we are just beginning to understand. Every day there is more to know about our physical ability to engage and manage the experiences of Second Adulthood.

Another research frontier particularly relevant to understanding the reinvention process of Second Adulthood is the relatively new academic discipline of gender studies. After thirty years of activism against stereotypical gender distinctions, the playing field has become level enough to begin looking at the real behavioral differences between men and women without imposing restrictions or value judgments on them. Sociologists, psychologists, political scientists, and feminists are exploring those traits, be they nurtured or natural, that take women and men down different roads to the same goal. A wide range of studies are analyzing the way men and women deal with moral questions, with power, and with the demands of daily life. Early analysis suggests that women's multifaceted thinking process and more improvisational approach to problem-solving are particularly suited to the challenges of Second Adulthood—not to mention the twenty-first-century world.

My current favorite example is how women and men deal with stress (that is, the modern-day form of danger once represented by a menacing jungle predator). We have always been taught that the human animal is equipped with a *fight-or-flight* response in which adrenaline mobilizes the body for enhanced speed to escape or enhanced strength to strike out. It turns out that those conclusions were drawn from studies done on men. According to University of California at Los Angeles (UCLA) psychologist Shelley E. Taylor, it is now clear that "every man for himself" is primarily a male response; women exhibit what scientists have labeled *tend-and-befriend* behavior. Our impulse in times of danger is to join with others in our group to make peace, to reach out to friend and foe, to defuse the situation. The genesis of the inquiry into women's behavior came, appropriately, in a casual girl talk between Taylor and her colleague Dr. Laura Cousino Klein. "There was this joke that when the women who worked in the lab were stressed, they came in, cleaned the lab, had coffee, and bonded," recalls Dr. Klein. "When the men were stressed, they holed up somewhere on their own." Their study is the result of their determination to find out why.

The notion that women seek safety in a social network is confirmed in animal studies. Another UCLA study found that while crowding made male rats more stressed, it calmed the females. An important source of this different behavior is the pituitary hormone oxytocin—best known for its role in labor before birth and lactation afterward—which has a calming effect and is produced in both men and women. The difference is that in men the effect of oxytocin—also known as the *hormone of love* or the *cuddle chemical*—is diminished by the release of testosterone, which promotes aggressive responses.

There is an interesting corollary to this discovery. Previous research shows that when adrenaline is rushing, as in the fight-or-flight response, cognitive functions are focused on the body's mobilization against danger. But those rational faculties are actually enhanced in a calmed-down state, which the tend-and-befriend mode is, and they can be called upon to think through a problem rather than attack or flee it.

These insights also offer a new perspective on women's friendships, which play an enhanced and crucial role in Second Adulthood. The network of friends we instinctively turn to is more than a support group; it is a significant survival technique. Not only because women are hard-wired to confront adversity better in groups, but because the combination of trust and respect we practice with each other is a model for the new intimacy that our changing circumstances call for in our other relationships.

The importance of this bond was confirmed by how often the women I have interviewed say that it was their friends that talked them through a crisis and, in general, kept them going. "I don't know what I would do without my friends" is a mantra we all chant. Few men have that kind of intimate support network; that may be one reason why they become less adventurous than women in Second Adulthood and why many seem to be going through a second *child*hood instead.

Women arrive at the frontier of this new stage with impressive credentials. Although we are flying under the radar, obscured by the wildly flawed expectation that we will become less and less who we were as we get older, we are poised to take off into the unknown. Futurist Ken Dychtwald, a consultant on what he calls the *age wave,* issued an early warning alert to a group of business executives about "the most amazing women our country has ever seen. They are living the most complex lives, managing households, managing jobs, dealing with in-laws. . . . We haven't come close to understanding the complexity of the mind, heart, and soul of these women" who, he added, "are going to become the power group in our country!"

The Journey

So, we are a new kind of generation. At the same time each of us is a new woman to herself. No wonder the journey begins in a torrent of confusion. Many women find themselves at the edge of the cliff before they even realize something is happening. And looking down, they can't imagine what ropes and pulleys will guide their descent.

They are propelled only by a funny feeling—like the first inkling of pregnancy. It is a mixture of dissatisfaction and fear—and a panicky sense that it is time to *do something.* Sooner or later each of us does do something. The *something* is different for every woman I talked to, as minor as throwing out that pillowcase full of mismatched socks once and for all, or as major as interviewing for a new job, getting divorced, or going back to school. But in each case, the ripples set off by those first almost random acts move out into unexpected corners of their lives. In the course of Second Adulthood every aspect of our being—our intimate relationships and our public selves, our professional commitments and our secret dreams, our drives and our fears—will be washed by those ripples; some may even be washed away. But the momentum that has been generated, disorienting as it might be, is driving us toward a wider horizon. As my friend Elizabeth reassures me when I feel atomized by the centrifugal force of events in my life, "a person who isn't expanding is a person who is contracting."

Since my week in the wilderness, I have switched careers, though not entirely by my own choosing. I have endured the tumultuous adolescence of my son while on the alarmingly parallel track of menopause. I lost twenty-five pounds (and, alas, gained a few back) and have begun to work out in a gym for the first time in my life. I have become a feisty big-mouth, in stark contrast to the conciliatory smoother-over of my first fifty years. I have undertaken the renegotiation of a thirty-five year marriage. I have made as many sardonic jokes as anyone about sagging flesh and memory lapses. And I am still trying to figure out how I am going to cross the shifting tectonic plates that lie between who I have been in my assimilated roles of daughter, friend, employee, wife, mother—and who I am becoming as I tap into my inner resources.

To illuminate my own journey and to clarify the promise and pitfalls of this stage of life, I have asked practically every woman I encountered over the past two years to tell me about her life at this moment in time. Even the experts I was consulting about their research dropped their professional distance once I explained what I was writing about and shared their personal expertise as well. Each is in the midst of her journey. Their stories are as worn around the edges as yours and mine. They have no neat endings or surefire tricks to offer; in most, the plot line meanders and doubles back and even disappears for a time. There are highs and lows. When I talked to them, some were euphoric because I caught them on a day when they had glimpsed a light at the end of a tunnel or when some piece had finally fallen into place or when they were simply having a good day. Others were feeling lost, desperately searching for a pattern, for a game plan.

But everyone found our conversation a rare opportunity to share personal discoveries, connect with what other women were experiencing, and take strength from that. And I'm sure you know how that strength expressed itself. Not in choruses of "I am woman, hear me roar!" but in laughter, our secret weapon. I cannot imagine getting through the day, let alone Second Adulthood—or this book, for that matter—without an ascerbic "are you ready for this?" from a friend or a hysterical dead-on observation about forgetfulness in an e-mail or a collective guffaw with my best once-a-month dinner friends over one of aging's absurdities. I would never leave home on any kind of journey without the friends I laugh with. They, along with the women I interviewed, and you the reader, are on this adventure with me. By sharing information and telling the truth, we will figure things out together.

So, with the understanding that this is a process and not a program, I can assure you of two things: you are not alone, and the trip will definitely be worth it.

An Itinerary

However much of the statistically projected quarter of a century any of us actually does get, it will be spent wrestling with The Question *(what am I going to do with the rest of my life?)* in its serial form—*what matters? what works?* and *what's next?* If I am not who I was, we inquire with apprehension, who am I now? Who do I want to become? How do I get there? What will that person make of her days?

The answers are different for every woman and even for the same women at different points along the way. In many ways, Second Adulthood is a mystery cruise to an undisclosed destination in wildly unpredictable weather, calling on ports dangerous and idyllic. And while The Question may drive the ship, the answer for many of us will lie not in a particular harbor but in the journey itself.

If it was possible to chart the journey in a formulaic way, it would go something like this: The You're-Not-Who-You-Were, Only-Older phase is totally discombobulating. Not only do you not know what is happening to you, but you don't even know what words will come out of your mouth next. You may hear yourself accept an invitation you were sure you would decline; or, instead of abjectly apologizing for a misstep, you hear yourself simply acknowledge it and move on. My early encounter with the euphoria of saying no is characteristic of the surge of defiance many women experience at first.

The confusion that results from such inappropriate and out-of-character behavior—the sense of falling—eventually gives way to a floating sensation in a gravity-free zone I call the Fertile Void. That is where we begin the process of sorting things out—and shaking things up. We shed the voices of shoulda-woulda-coulda thinking and begin to sense the presence of an internal compass, our own voice. With its guidance, we can zero in on our personal truth—to distinguish between the fire of an authentic drive and the drone of automatic pilot. Little by little, we get in touch with that elusive essential—our passions.

Emboldened by these important discoveries about ourselves, we enter the *recalibration* phase. There we become engaged in the delicate business of revising our priorities and renegotiating our relationships. This is when we look at our worklife and our love life and take stock of our circumstances. Initially, most of us think the decisions we need to make about the future are practical ones, along the lines of changing jobs or taking up woodworking, making to-do lists and cleaning out closets, but

the Fertile Void soul searching reveals that we are really confronting multiple versions of The Question. Some versions are
metaphysical, some practical, some emotional: How do I take
care of my body for the rest of my life? How will I manage my
finances? What activities will make me feel productive and
successful? How do I cope with adversity? And, most painfully:
How do I love? There is nothing harder than trying to convince a bewildered partner or child that you are discovering
new ways of loving them. But we are.

As the pieces of self-knowledge and self-determination begin to fall into place, what at first appeared to be a chaotic and
sometimes fool-hardy enterprise morphs into a more philosophical and authoritative frame of mind, a phase I call *making
peace and taking charge.* This is when we implement some changes
and begin to believe that we can handle whatever life throws at
us. At this point it becomes inviting to look beyond the limits
of our inner voices and our immediate concerns—to the
world around us. Some women become galvanized by community activities or go back to school; others take a new look
at the impact of their work or at the spiritual component in
their lives. Many are drawn to the generations ahead or behind
them and come to feel more grounded in the human family.

Ideally—which means rarely—these stages build upon each
other so that a sense of mastery meets the riptides set off by the
painful, and invigorating, and inevitable business of recalibrating every gauge in our lives. For most of us, though, it seems to
be happening all at once. Still, with every risk we take, we become more confident that we can cope with and even embrace
conflict and change. And as we meet the challenges described
in the chapters that follow, the discoveries we make about our
inner resources empower us to take on the next one.

MARGO'S STORY
There's Just No Static on the Line

You will meet many complex and exciting women in the pages that follow, but I do want to introduce you now to Margo (whose name, like some of the others in this book, has been changed to protect her privacy). Her story struck me as a paradigm for the Second Adulthood process. Margo's husband died twelve years before we met and her two sons had only recently moved on into their own lives. For thirty years, Margo, now fifty-five, had worked as a high-powered corporate executive and had relished the excitement her career brought. But suddenly, she was feeling claustrophobic, a condition many women experience in widely differing forms. "I felt my world was small and getting smaller," she told me. Margo was bewildered. "I had always had a lot of ambition and aggression. And then I didn't. What happened?"

As she continued to push herself to meet the job demands that used to feel like a welcome challenge, she tested out alternatives. Since she'd always loved antiques, she thought she might try being a buyer for other dealers, but a few courses in antiques convinced her she "didn't want to go back to school," and several months scrounging flea markets convinced her that she couldn't earn a living as a "picker." She tried to push her imagination further; she even "thought it might be fun to be a character actor in commercials. But," Margo concludes, "one by one, I eliminated all those ideas."

Then serendipity struck. A young woman her son was dating was about to leave for the Peace Corps, and everything she described about that program sounded just right. Margo, the urban executive; Margo, whose lifelong hobby—around which she planned her busy schedule—was ballet classes; Margo, the driven, bossy, power broker; *that very Margo* found herself a year later in a tiny village in the Ivory Coast, speaking fluent French and designing latrine-building projects. What does Margo say about all this? "I have no idea why I had so little trouble adjusting. There is just no static on the line!" What a glorious prospect: a stage of life that brings clarity, confidence, and purpose!

But her journey doesn't stop there. In a couple of years Margo plans to come home and become a consultant on economic development to international corporations. And lest anyone think she's thrown over her old self altogether, she expects to pick up ballet again (though a few classes when she came home for the birth of her first grandchild showed her that she "couldn't do a turned-out plié as gracefully as before"). And she intends to make the most of her new self. "I have a nest egg," she explains, "but I do need to earn money. I'm used to earning and dressing and being and going—being chic. You can't do that on a fixed income. Maintenance is expensive. Being a jazzy older woman costs money. And that includes plastic surgery—when I get back from the Peace Corps."

Margo and you and I are the first generation of women nurtured on a recognition of women's independence; that gives us the chutzpah to go for a Second Adulthood. We are the first generation to be recipients of new levels of health and longevity expectations; that gives us the time for a Second Adulthood. We are the largest segment of the largest population demographic in U.S. history, and that gives us consumer and political clout to shape a new social experience called Second Adulthood. And science is producing breakthrough research showing brain changes that suggest our outlook is literally being redesigned from the inside; that gives us affirmation for what we are finding out about Second Adulthood.

What we don't have yet are role models or road maps for the journey, and that can make freedom feel like chaos, and promise feel like wishful thinking. I offer the brain research news, sketchy as it is, as a metaphor for Second Adulthood. If a woman looks at what is happening to her as a learning curve of her new brain power, she will be more receptive to the impulse to reconsider her experience, revisit her decisions, and reorganize her emotions. Willing to step off the cliff and meet the not-yet-known.

Like our first adulthood, Second Adulthood begins with a turbulent adolescence.

Second Adolescence

A Second Chance at Growing Up Strong

When Sleeping Beauty wakes up, she is almost fifty years old.

—Maxine Kumin

As we enter our fifties, many women who, like me, postponed having children, find themselves going through menopause around the same time their children are going through adolescence. In my case, my daughter began to menstruate just as I was beginning to miss periods; and my son was well on his way to becoming a master at talking back by the time I hit my Outward Bound no! epiphany. The physiological hits of menopause left me relatively unscathed, but I met up with the who-am-I-and-where-am-I-going demons of Second Adulthood just as my son was encountering his own adolescent version of those same demons. Juxtaposing the two life passages has helped me see that both are launching pads into the future. My teenagers and I are grappling with the same two disorienting questions: What is happening to my body? and Who am I?

What's Happening to Me?

Raging hormones. We have hot flashes, teenagers have acne. We stop menstruating, they begin. We sleep less, they sleep more. We lose libido, theirs goes bonkers. They grow hair, ours thins. Both age groups are prone to extreme mood swings and strange behavior. When I complained to the father of five grown children about my son's unpredictable ways, he smiled knowingly and explained that I would have to accept that a teenager simply becomes a "werewolf" for a while—an unrecognizable creature of the night. The description struck me. It wasn't so long ago that a woman going through the change of life was also considered a werewolf of sorts, an unbalanced harpy in a constant state of PMS, who literally changed color and grew fur without warning.

The major difference is that the teenage werewolf is accepted as a stage of life, while the menopausal werewolf is considered an affliction in need of treatment. In my mother's generation, doctors prescribed tranquilizers to tame the beast. Husbands and media wits told jokes about her. Then, beginning in the 1980s, doctors had a new treatment—hormone replacement therapy (HRT). In addition to subduing many physiological symptoms, it allayed anxiety and promoted a sense of well-being and energy for some women. Since then, some fifteen million women a year have begun hormone therapy; in 1999 alone, ninety million prescriptions were written.

Recent alarming findings have forced us to make some tough choices (see Chapter Nine). In 2002, the National Institutes of Health halted a major clinical trial of an HRT drug because of an increase in the incidence of breast cancer among its participants. But many women have been reluctant to give up the boost HRT gives. A woman gynecologist I consulted is among them. "Postmenopausal women have more power today than ever before," she began. "Why do anything that will reduce that power and energy unless there is a strong medical reason for that particular patient? I know what estrogen is doing for me. I wouldn't be working at such a high level and enjoying it so much if I went off estrogen. Sure it's a risk, but I ski and that is a risk too."

The debate goes on. We will have to await new studies of Second Adulthood women to determine what role, if any, replacing the estrogen that launched us into puberty can play in our relaunch. In addition hormone research on adolescents may turn up other relevant findings. For example, reduced levels of the mood-enhancing hormone serotonin in teenagers have been cited as sources of both depression and impulsiveness. Though menopausal women, who are known to suffer bouts of depression, have yet to be studied in the same way, the documented fluctuations in that hormone may explain something about the out-of-character behavior we are experiencing, too.

Overall, looking at our werewolf behavior as a rerun of the scary movie adolescence is acknowledged to be enables us to see our rebellious behavior for what it is—a physical, psychological, and emotional shake-up that announces our Second Adulthood, a transition into a promising new stage of understanding and accomplishment.

Brain Waves

Even our brains are maturing in ways that promote this transition. Recent research shows for the first time that we and adolescents—and no other age group—experience new brain growth. It takes place in the medial temporal lobe, the area identified with emotional learning. The actual new growth is in myelin, the fatty coating to nerve fibers that insulates and speeds up connections between nerve cells. This augmented brain activity plays a crucial role in helping us synthesize what experience teaches, and it enhances our ability to make considered judgment calls. As I see it, the same process that accounts for the transformation of impulsive and irresponsible teenagers into thoughtful adults comes back for an encore at midlife, just in time to make us even more thoughtful—dare I say wise? Overall, I find it reassuring to conclude that if I seem to not be myself lately, I can chalk it up to my newly greased synapses playing with the new me.

Dr. Francine Benes, a fifty-six-year-old professor of psychiatry at Harvard Medical School, was the first to document this brain activity. When she began, she had no intention of finding the neurochemistry of Second Adulthood. She had been studying the genesis of schizophrenia, which often manifests itself in adolescence, by analyzing cross sections of 160 male and female brains of all ages, looking for something that might happen to teenagers that would trigger the disease. Coming upon the myelination growth spurt, she prepared to report her discovery to the scientific community and thought a graph would make her information clearer. To make the spike in the graph as dramatic as possible, she decided to extend it over the entire age range she had studied. That was when she saw the second spike.

The graph showed two significant increases in the accumulation of myelin: a 100 percent growth during the teenage years and another 50 percent (a "*huge*" jump, she says) around age fifty. Since then others have made similar observations using brain-imaging techniques on live subjects. Another interesting finding from Dr. Benes's research is that the myelination growth spurt occurred much earlier and faster in girls and was almost complete by the end of middle school. The surge of estrogen at the same time is thought to be responsible for the faster growth in another part of the adolescent girl's brain, the

hippocampus, which is where memory, a key to social maturation, is developed. For boys there is a significant lag behind
girls in brain development; the maturation process can extend
past the teenage years into the twenties. This pattern suggests
that in both brain development and behavior, maturity begins
earlier in the life cycle for women. Furthermore, not only have
women been socialized earlier—and, therefore, experienced
the challenges of adolescence from a different perspective—
but, as we well know, we have been socialized differently. So,
while the second shot of brain growth is the same in men and
women and occurs around the same age, men do not come
into their fifties with the same social history that we do. They
experience hormonal changes, too, but not the major hormonal, psychological, and social upheaval of menopause. Un-
doubtedly, they will respond to the brain changes differently.

Emotions

Adolescence is notorious for its emotionality. And changes in
our brain chemistry impact the way we assimilate emotional
experience, or, more precisely, how we process *feelings*—which
we are generating apace throughout Second Adulthood. Neuroscientist Antonio Damasio (at the University of Iowa Medical Center and author of *The Feeling of What Happens*) is
pioneering a new understanding of the interdependence of
emotion and reason. Emotions, he explains, are the first reaction to an experience and they are largely physiological. They
are "public and can be seen," he says. "You can see me crying
or getting angry but," he goes on, "you can never see what I
am experiencing when I am feeling angry, happy, or sad."
Those are feelings, which affect a different part of the brain
from emotions, and they are "private, internal, and personal."

How we incorporate those feelings throughout our lives has important implications for the person we become. We call upon them throughout our lives, Damasio explains, for "planning, anticipation, and decision making." Those "stored feelings" also enable us "to empathize with people experiencing the same feelings." The impetus of accumulated empathy at our stage of life may be a source of our willingness to take on fearsome foes; as psychiatrist Jean Shinoda Bolen puts it, in her book *Crones Don't Whine,* "The suffering of others or the feeling of *enough is enough* radicalizes older women."

As stored feelings bubble up and radical impulses are generated during Second Adulthood, we find ourselves revisiting ideas and experiences gathered over a lifetime. Things are adding up in new ways. Some women report a sudden loss of interest in the past. "I'm sick of saving things," one woman told me, "including resentments. I quit therapy recently because I didn't want to look back any more. I just want to move on." Others want to do just the opposite—to use their newfound feistiness to tell off historic bullies and clarify longstanding misunderstandings. "I see patterns now," says Mary. "And they explain so many events that I thought came out of the blue. That helps me look ahead."

We are sometimes overwhelmed by the emotional turmoil of reviewing our relationships, reevaluating ourselves, and wondering who we will be when we grow up. Just like teenagers. There is a difference, though, between how we deal with this heady brew at our later stage of life and how they react. "Adolescents are very emotive, very responsive to external stimuli, very excitable," says Dr. Benes. "As we mature we become more focused and more in command of our emotions. There's a greater calmness that comes during midlife." Her words suggest to me a scheme of things in which the early myelination works to help the brain tame the wild, primitive emotions that we are born with. The second time around it heightens the synthesis of what we've learned and felt since adolescence.

Dr. Benes speculates that this brain activity may explain why, as psychologists have observed, distressing qualities we have been living with—such as anxiety, the need to be accepted by the crowd, and the experience of being thrown by events—are modified with age. We become more inwardly directed and are more inclined to enjoy our own company. Even though the stresses and disappointments of aging are real, we seem to be more philosophical about them, unlike adolescents who tend to catastrophize even the smallest misadventure. A recent study by psychologist David Almeida (at the University of Arizona at Tucson) found that among one thousand adults over twenty-five, only 8 percent of the young adults reported one stress-free day out of eight, in contrast to 12 percent of those forty to fifty-nine and 19 percent of those over sixty. "The older you get," he concludes, "you kind of realize that 'hey, it's not worth getting upset about the small things.'"

Making peace with the inevitability of bumps in the road—what many women I talked to described as a newfound "mellowness"—does not arrive with the immediacy of a hot flash. It isn't always there when you need it, but it does accumulate along the way. There is a poetic irony in the notion that the term associated with the blissed-out hippie of an earlier era in our lives has come around again in connection with a laid-back pragmatist.

Obviously such sweeping changes in our outlook are not entirely due to the myelination in our brains. But they confirm that, as Dr. Benes put it, "with improved nutrition and exercise and overall good health, our brains are *not* programmed to deteriorate." One cannot assume, she concludes, that "improvement in our ability to manage our emotions is related to brain development alone. Cumulative experience is contributing in a very substantive way to making us the individuals we are." One *can* assume, however, that what is going on "changes the way one thinks about oneself." Psychologically as well as physically, we are *not* who we were, only older.

Who Am I?

In adolescence it is called an identity crisis, and solving it is considered the main psychological work of that stage. In Second Adulthood, the way one thinks about oneself is just as crucial. As we evaluate our experience so far and contemplate the possibilities ahead—as we wrestle with The Question—we meet our sense of self with an intensity that we may not have experienced for thirty or forty years. Changes that take place in that crucible, and the way we recalibrate our lives in response to them, result in a personality shake-up. Every woman I spoke with was struggling to get to know herself anew. The stirrings of introspection that accompany the other emotional, neurological, and hormonal shifts of second adolescence become more insistent as we move ahead.

For the average woman, focusing on her self has been a furtive business at best. The education process for women of our age has been in pleasing, caring for, and empathizing with others. Even when she was wielding power or earning money, a women often felt she had to first factor in the needs of those around her. Urged to take one day a month to pamper herself, or take to heart the airline safety instruction to put her oxygen mask on before attending to her children, she has been reluctant to accept such counterintuitive advice. The first cover of *Ms.* magazine in 1972 was a drawing of a blue Shiva-like woman with eight arms, each holding a tool of her trade—a mop, a baby bottle, a typewriter. It resonated with thousands of women who were going crazy trying to do it all. I see that figure as an energy field that is being depleted—a generic woman with thousands of tiny arrows all pointing outward, from her brain, her hands, her heart, her genitals—a sort of St. Sebastian in reverse. With so much energy exiting the system throughout our first adulthood, it has been hard to hold onto enough to turn the focus inward.

Yet that is precisely what we want and need to do in our Second Adulthood. One of the most profound psychological shifts that takes place as we move into that new stage is a reversal of the caretaking system: we begin to hear one another say "I'm going to take better care of myself." By that we mean more than getting an occasional massage—though pampering is on the agenda. We mean listening more closely to the needs and passions we have shunted aside because we were *too busy*. At the same time we are tuning out some of those demands that kept us so busy. "It is such a relief," says Amy, who is only weeks away from retirement, "to hear myself saying, 'That's not my problem; let someone else take care of it.' I am looking forward to taking care of *myself*."

Alexis, a recently retired gym teacher, is just beginning to readjust. "It used to be like everything I did was other-directed—teaching for others, mothering for others, being a wife. Now with retiring I feel like I'm so self-oriented; I guess I still feel a sense of apology about focusing on myself; it's very difficult to make that leap."

Despite the centrifugal forces that have beset us, each of us has always been aware—however dimly—of an inner life. We've sheltered it from outside demands by a second skin that protects a closed system of conversations inside one's head, intimacies exchanged only with friends, or thoughts jotted down in secret journals. But the protective membrane has, over the years, become hardened to leather. As we spend more quality time with our buried self, we also begin to experience the satisfaction that comes from within.

Ellen has a full life. She is the director of a major organization and speaks in public on policy issues. She is also the mother of two grown children and the wife of an artist whose studio takes up half of the converted barn they live in. A chance series of events gave Ellen the opportunity for a personal synthesis of two aspects of her creative life that had been on parallel tracks. As a photography buff as well as an administrator, she often took photographs to accompany the studies generated by her company. Some of the research involved children at play, and her images added an important dimension to the reports. Far away, on the other side of her life, Ellen and her family spent several summers in a remote mountain village on a Greek island that was literally being washed away. "For the past eighteen years I have been photographing the deterioration," she says. "It is so eerie and beautiful to see nature reclaiming the tiny village we live in and so poignant to watch the population fade away." Those have been her private photographs, the ones she keeps in boxes at home.

One day, she showed a neighbor in her suburban community one of her Greek photographs that she had framed; he had just become director of a local arts center and was looking for material to exhibit. He liked the Greek series but felt they were not enough for a one-woman show. "Do you have anything else?" he asked. "No," replied Ellen. "Wait a minute!" said her husband. "What about the children playing stuff?" "But that's about work," Ellen protested. She couldn't imagine showing her professionally detached reportage alongside her personal exploration of nature and decay. If anything, it would be a *two-woman* show. The director prevailed, and Ellen was in agony anticipating the opening when people who only know the professional side would get a glimpse of her secret self. But when she looked around the gallery she saw Ellen-the-photographer, whole for the first time.

Psychologist Carol Gilligan, who first studied the lost voice of adolescent girls and the disconnect between their inner life and public behavior, turned, in her recent book, *The Birth of Pleasure*, to the process of repairing the disassociation between "a cover story and an under-reality." Like many of the experts I consulted about Second Adulthood, Gilligan responded by drawing on details of her own life. Her experience shows that, for women of our generation, awareness—even at the highest level—is not enough; the circumstances have to change—which they do in Second Adulthood. Now sixty-eight, she has only just begun to explore new aspects of her talents. After decades of publishing clinical analyses of her subjects' experience, she is—to her great joy—focusing her imagination and her own experience to a novel. This could not have happened, she told me, before the last of her three sons got married when she was in her fifties. Only then did she feel liberated from the "box" which, in a recurrent dream, symbolized the home she tended for her family. Now she has begun to dream outside the intellectual box she had constructed.

Trudy is high on self-discovery, too. The exhilaration she describes differs only in style—and perhaps intensity—from what so many women told me they felt as they began to know themselves. A lifelong rebel, activist, and poet, she has been a marijuana smoker for years; she had used it socially, to enhance conversation, humor, and sex. But recently getting high has become a totally inner-directed experience. "I turn on when I am alone and begin to feel a wave of joy, joy in myself. I leave notes for myself on the refrigerator that I find the next morning: 'I really *like* you,' or 'you will get through this,'" she says with a smile. (She also finds, to her dismay, that the house is under a blanket of cookie crumbs and stray popcorn bits, the byproduct of one thing that hasn't changed about getting stoned—"the awful munchies.")

In adolescence, we struggle to capture elusive shards of personality and make them our own; in second adolescence the challenge is to excavate some of those shards from the buried compartments they have been consigned to. The drive to synthesize past and present, inner life and public self, energizes the future with the promise of a growing sense of integrity, authenticity, and uniqueness. When Sleeping Beauty awakens at fifty, she's done with fairy tales and ready to write her own—in her own voice.

VIVI'S STORY
"The Choices I'm Making Are Much More Personal and Quiet"

Vivi, a computer programmer, is just getting used to a revised relationship with herself that began as she entered her fifties. "I'm a single woman and I've always been very active in community work, in volunteer work. . . . Three years ago, I would have said, 'Yes, I'm vibrantly involved and connected and participating,' which I was. Then something changed for me, and I sort of dropped out of all that and became just a private person."

Vivi is the daughter of Holocaust survivors who emigrated to the United States. In her twenties, she moved to Israel and married there; she became a farmer, because that was what her husband wanted to do. "I gave up everything—my work, my city life . . . because I was very much in love." But with an enthusiasm that is one of her most noteworthy traits, she said to herself, "Okay, we'll try this." And to her surprise she "wound up loving it"—more, it turns out, than she ended up loving her husband. When the marriage broke up, she left the country and the life she had built there. Back in the United States, she had a hard time finding a job. When someone suggested she study data processing, characteristically (again) she gave it a try. "It was very hard for me because that kind of work was contrary to my nature, but I had to support myself." That's how she ended up with a bifurcated lifestyle—divided between "the things I earn my living at and the things that are my passions. I wish," she adds wistfully, "that I could have been paid for my passions—community building, travel, adventure."

The "corporate world" where she continues to work "is not a pretty place," she said. "You're treated not as an individual person with certain skills that are valued. You're treated as a sort of plug-n-play resource." In fact, she has never even met many of the people she works with. "It's all telephone conferences . . . just voices you learn to recognize." Concerned about holding onto that financial base, last year she subjected herself to a six-week course in a distant city to update her skills. "I realized that I couldn't keep coasting on the skills I had, but it was so exhausting to my brain. I hated every minute."

While her practical life was uninspiring but on track, events in her other life were forcing Vivi to look inward. She had been a founding member of an alternative synagogue, but as the congregation became more established, it became more impersonal. "The institution just changed direction in a way which wasn't meaningful to me," she explains. She struggled on until she realized she had undergone an "evolution" from "big commitment to no commitment." And she "dropped out."

Dropping out became "a moment in time to reevaluate and

make other choices," a perfect description of the stage I call the Fertile Void, the subject of the next chapter. As she looked at the forces that were propelling her there, a pattern emerged that many women recognize and psychologists' observations reinforce: we become more introspective with age. "In general," says Vivi, "the choices I am making are much more personal and quiet and involve less people . . . I don't want as many people around . . . and that makes it hard in terms of friendships that have kind of traveled with you. Perhaps the wave that carries them is nostalgia, because you've been together for so long. You don't want to lose those relationships . . . but I'm finding that I need a lot of away time, quiet time. Many people don't understand why I'm so comfortable being alone. But I don't really feel lonely."

Vacations became increasingly important to Vivi, and are now "a kind of holy time." She is grateful to have a like-minded friend who shares her interest in off-beat destinations. When we spoke, she had just returned from hiking and biking in Nova Scotia. The year before she and her traveling companion got to Land's End in England. No one could understand why they chose such a godforsaken spot. "When you are there," she enthuses, "it is just so magnificent, the roar of the ocean against the mountains, against the rocks . . . those are the kind of places that speak to me."

As we enter Second Adulthood, each of us is poised at a Land's End of our own, looking out over an elemental and unruly terrain. We are only just beginning to understand where we are capable of going from here. One thing we do know, thanks to recent discoveries about the brain, is that we will have our faculties with us. But we also recognize the need to travel light. In the same way that we lose memory but gain insight, much of the business of this transition requires making do with less. The identity we shape in our second adolescence will reflect the wisdom with which we make peace with what was—and what is.

As Vivi described how much she gave up when she moved to the desert farm she came to love, she evoked the journey into the desert of sorts that we are all embarking on. "I'd always been a city person, so how could I go to a place that didn't have green and didn't have trees and didn't have the kind of smell and the kind of sounds that I was familiar with? It's such a different rhythm of life." Then she explained how she had engaged the experience. "You have to look at the desert with desert eyes. You can't bring your city eyes to the desert—or you'll be very disappointed. If you look out of your desert eyes, you see amazing things that are there."

———

When I first read that psychiatrist Elisabeth Kübler-Ross had called adolescence "the birth of the soul," I thought it was an apt metaphor. Now, as I listen to Vivi's words and consider the parallels between us and our teenagers, I see the phrase has a powerful validity for Second Adulthood, too. The Question is as much about how we know our soul as it is about how we fill our time. As we begin to adjust to the notion that we are not who we were, only older, we can imagine that what life is offering us is a chance to experience the *re*birth of the soul.

CHAPTER THREE

Defiance

Speaking Up,
Speaking Out, Speaking Your Mind

Age 3: She looks at herself and sees a queen.
Age 8: She looks at herself and sees Cinderella.
Age 15: She looks at herself and sees an Ugly Sister and says, "Mom, I can't go to school looking like this!"
Age 20: She looks at herself and sees "too fat/too thin, too short/too tall, too straight/too curly"—but decides she's going out anyway.
Age 30: She looks at herself and sees "too fat/too thin, too short/too tall, too straight/too curly"—but decides she doesn't have time to fix it so she's going out anyway.
Age 40: She looks at herself and sees "too fat/too thin, too short/too tall, too straight/too curly"—but says, "At least I'm clean" and goes out anyway.
Age 50: She looks at herself and sees "I am" and goes wherever she wants to go.

—anonymous lines circulated on the Internet with a note to pass it on to "all the women you are grateful to have as friends."

Adolescents have numerous rites of passage—becoming a teen-ager, getting a driver's license, religious confirmation, graduation, voting for the first time—and adulthood has its share, but over the course of a life, except for funerals, they peter out. Even birthdays lose their luster. As my friends and I inched past forty, we would keep quiet about the date. If someone happened to remember, the protocol was to ask coyly if it is "a round number." Now more and more of us are reclaiming fifty, albeit with misgivings and incredulity, but also with defiance.

Some women have given themselves just the kind of party they always wanted. "If I can't do what I want at fifty," one woman explained in her "noninvitations" to friends, children, and husband, "when can I do it?" She told them that she wanted to be alone on that day, but would like to receive letters from each of them as a birthday gift. She spent the day spontaneously going to museums, getting her hair cut, giving a fifty—get it?—dollar bill to a street musician, and reading those heartfelt testimonials. "It was the perfect rite of passage" she recalls. "For me." Others have been dragged kicking and screaming to a girls' night out or a spa day. For my birthday, it was my husband who insisted on an event. I squirmed at the idea, but now I am extremely grateful. Everyone was asked to bring a photo of themselves taken at the time I came into their lives. Many had photos of the two of us together—in camp, in high school, in the office. The photo album of that night includes those snapshots as well as photos of our more shopworn selves taken at the party. It is a treasure.

Several women commemorated their milestone with a meaningful act. Some went out and cut their hair short. Others quit smoking. Whether we claim the birthday or try to brush it under the rug, whether we find ourselves becoming curious about the future or depressed over the past, we understand instinctively that we need to mark the stirrings of change we feel.

A fiftieth birthday becomes a marker of that precarious moment we find ourselves in—the tipping point between who we were until now and who we are about to become. It is our graduation from first adulthood. Gestalt psychologist Fritz Perls made the simple but profound observation that maturity is the process of moving from dependency on the environment to dependency on the self. We were daughters, mothers, partners, employees, and each of those titles brought with it a time-tested script of its own. We may carry these relationships with us into Second Adulthood, but we are done with the roles that came with them. Each of us is now writing her own script. In her own voice.

Speaking up, speaking out, speaking one's mind—these are all attributes of Second Adulthood that each woman I interviewed experienced. In acts large and small we are standing up for ourselves—telling off the patronizing salesperson, taking an unpopular position at a dinner table debate, confronting a bullying spouse. "I just don't care what people think anymore!" is the universal and amazed refrain. But it's more subtle and profound than that. In her memoir *Saturday's Child,* Robin Morgan writes about discovering "that it's not that I no longer care what other people think. I do care, actually. It's simply that I finally care more what *I* think." I call it The Fuck You Fifties.

The Big No

Most of our acts of rebellion—like my refusing to climb back up the face of that cliff in Maine—have to do with saying no. No, I don't want to listen to that music. No, I don't want to spend an evening with that bore. No, I don't want to look like that. No, I don't want to help. . . . Before we can affirm who we are, we have to say *no* to some long-held assumptions about who we are. Am I the nice, responsible "fabulous kid" I have tried to sell myself as since high school, I wonder, or am I the somewhat more mean-spirited and slightly slothful soul I now recognize—and like hanging out with a whole lot better?

Until I got feisty, I kept my voice low and listened for the signals from the outside that would answer a different set of questions: Will they like me? Will they approve of what I am doing? What do they need from me? You may wonder who "they" are—I wish I knew. The judgmental "they" was everyone else—including, I once admitted to a shocked friend, my children. For the most part I hid this anxious-to-please mouse. I made tough decisions, I expressed opinions, I held my head up. But that posture often felt like just another role—that of a competent self-confident grown-up. It's been called the Impostor Syndrome—the secret suspicion that you are faking it, that you are not really as good at things as others think you are. I had drifted away from the lights of my own shore. Now, the more out of character I behave, the more waves I make, the more I feel those waves are propelling me home, to myself.

Individual acts of speaking up, talking back, and telling the truth have added up to some big changes in the way the world sees me and, most important, in the way I see myself in the world. I have begun to keep a list of the Things I Don't Do Anymore. They affirm that I am not who I was, only older.

I don't do ladylike. I don't wear any clothes—itchy wool, hobbling skirts, high-heel shoes—that I can't wait to get out of when I get home. I don't mind my manners. I don't want to be popular. In fact, there are certain people I consider it a badge of honor to be disliked by. I don't panic at the first disapproving look, condescending smirk, or sharp retort. I am ready to plunge into controversy and argue rather than make peace.

To my surprise this approach makes me kinder than being *nice* did. Because there are many occasions when what I had been stifling (to recall Archie Bunker's admonition to Edith) were arguments over things that mattered to me, but were dismissed as sentimental issues. Now I speak up for children and animals—and for kindness itself.

I don't tell my friends how to run their lives anymore. I have been dispensing advice for most of my adult life. I was so sure I knew best. And because I knew the rules so well, I didn't seek advice from others when I should have. Over the years, for example, I have advised countless people to quit their unhappy jobs. To my secret contempt, not one has done it. Then, when it was my turn to contemplate an untenable work situation, it didn't take long before I developed both a profound empathy for their inertia and an intense interest in alternatives to all-or-nothing strategies. Not only have I stopped dispensing advice so cavalierly, I've stopped relying entirely on my own advice. What I might have lost in godliness, I've gained in . . . well, good advice.

I don't hold grudges anymore. Not just my own grudges—more than once I had banished someone from my holiday greetings list on behalf of a friend who had long since forgiven the offense. I've gotten tired of all that bookkeeping. Now when the friend who always cancels dates doesn't show up at the Weight Watchers meeting we vowed to attend as a team, I shrug—that's who she is—and move on.

I no longer hold onto things, either. I have thrown out truckloads of stuff, though I still have all my report cards from grade school, my diaries from teenage treks through Europe, the bouquet of ribbons from my bridal shower. But I haven't *added* anything new. I am less sentimental now. I think that is because I associate sentiment with nostalgia and loss, and that is not where I am right now. I'm into What's Next?

I don't take most things so seriously anymore. I've raised the bar on life-and-death crises. Arriving late, screwing up, or plans gone awry no longer qualify.

I don't, on the other hand, take some things so lightly. Especially sickness and danger. I have come to understand that I can't assume that every affliction is a prelude to recovery. That every close call won't get closer.

I don't make elaborate "to do" lists. I am hoping to liberate some of the energy I have invested in controlling things. Partly because in my first adulthood I learned that life is, as John Lennon put it, what happens when you are busy making other plans. And partly because in my Second Adulthood, I intend to travel light. I'm down to What Matters, What Works, and What's Next!

What *is* next? One thing is sure—there is no turning back. With each satisfaction, I believe that defiant and practical voice will get stronger. It will declare What Matters. It will clarify What Works. And that will prepare us for What's Next. But beyond that, as we move through this transition from dependence on the environment to dependence on ourselves, we find that what lies ahead is . . . more change.

Estrogen, Testosterone, and Healthy Anger

Along with big talk and outrageous behavior—or perhaps because of it—the Fuck You Fifties generates energy. Even among those who have problems with the psychological and physiological symptoms of menopause, there is recognition of what feminist Germaine Greer called "peaceful potency" and anthropologist Margaret Mead identified in all cultures she studied as "postmenopausal zest"—a stunning burst of energy and assertiveness. For all that is supposedly lost with the change of life, many women experience newfound personal freedom—and the energy to use it.

Current research shows that this surge is due in part to a hormonal reconfiguration that takes place. As estrogen goes down, testosterone—which has been there all along but held in check by the estrogen—begins to assert more influence. Though it, too, declines somewhat, the liberated testosterone produces varying degrees of male-like behavior—assertiveness, uninhibitedness, and spatial acuity (the ability to find your car in a parking lot), as well as the less appealing attributes of increased facial hair and thinning head hair.

The shifting estrogen-testosterone ratio also affects how we use our anger. Dr. Christiane Northrup, author of *The Wisdom of Menopause,* who has done more than almost anyone to redefine the transition, reports that changing levels of estrogen in the brain, particularly in the amygdala and hippocampus—areas where experience is transformed into memory and our most basic emotions are stored—"may well help to bring up old memories, accompanied by old emotions, especially anger." Anger is a touchy subject and a source of great ambivalence for many women. "Anger in women has a bad rap in general unless that anger arises in the service of others," Northrup points out. But "the political is always personal: our anger is ultimately about ourselves, and its energy is always urging us toward self-actualization." Emboldened by the Fuck You Fifties mindset, we are mobilizing to take on the personal offenses, social injustices, and disappointments that can still be turned around. "Using anger as a catalyst for positive change and growth is always liberating," Northrup concludes.

Another consequence of menopause is that our internal *biological clock* is reset to a more energy-efficient mode. The monthly cycle of buildup and letdown is replaced by an extended hum of activity. Getting off the hormonal roller coaster and onto the straightaway of one's own metabolism is a smoother ride. No longer at the mercy of a biological imperative, a woman is free to find her own rhythm. Being able to say "I'm taking *my* time now" is a declaration of independence.

Becoming Society's Free Radicals

Most liberating of all may be the release from the potential to get pregnant and everything that has meant in our lives: trying *not* to get pregnant; trying to *get* pregnant; feeling vulnerable to rape and other kinds of aggressive behavior; feeling "feminine" or not; feeling fulfilled or not; feeling valued or not.

Humans are the only species that experiences a midlife loss of fertility, and in many societies—although not our own—that is considered an attainment of status. "The native people say you don't become an adult until you are fifty-one," says Jyoti, who travels around the world studying indigenous cultures. "When you stop 'bleeding down' your wisdom stops going out. You begin to gather it. Then you have ten more years before you become a wise elder." The spiritual *gathering in* of resources that Joyti's words evoke—and so many women describe feeling this despite the turmoil of menopause—fuels the defiance that begins with the Fuck You Fifites and nurtures the sorting out process that follows.

Of all the women with whom I discussed menopause—most of whom confirmed the sense of relief it brought—the most enthusiastic welcome to the end of fertility came from a woman who I would have thought had the most to lose: a world-renowned model and actress whose sensuality and desirability had been her stock in trade. She underwent a hysterectomy just before her fiftieth birthday and, although she had dreaded everything about it, what she experienced was "a sense of liberation! It marked the end of my role as a possible sex object." From that day on, she told me, she became "more assertive." Letting go of that chapter in her life had freed her to say no to expectations not her own. "When I stopped being 'a woman' I could be what I wanted. I am not pleasing men or anyone. Only myself."

Anthropologist Kristen Hawkes is one of a new generation of scientists studying our species from the novel perspective of women's experience. She asks the question: what if nature has another assignment for us that takes advantage of our postmenopausal zest?

Hawkes lived with a tribe called the Hadza in northern Tanzania. On a typical day, the men are off hunting and the mothers are caring for numerous children. Hawkes realized that no one mother could gather enough food to feed multiple children on her own, particularly a nursing mother who requires six hundred more calories than usual for herself. So how do the toddlers survive? The free radicals in this situation are the no-longer-fertile women. They go where they are needed and take up the responsibility for tending to any needy children, not just their own grandchildren.

Hawkes concludes that evolution's purpose for women who are strong and healthy but beyond childbearing is to support the unique feature of human development—an extended childhood. During those protected years, the brain has time to grow into its complex human form and the community has time to teach intellectual and social skills to the next generation. Without supernumerary mothers, too many growing children would fall prey to natural dangers and the system would not have proved fit enough to survive.

The so-called grandmother effect is becoming a recognized evolutionary force. In 2002 the first international conference devoted to the role of the grandmother attracted evolutionary biologists, anthropologists, sociologists, and demographers from around the world. *New York Times* science writer Natalie Angier reported their overall conclusion: that grandmothers "have been an underrated source of power and sway in our evolutionary heritage." And a widely heralded study by Dr. Ronald Lee, a demographer at the University of California at Berkeley, found that "natural selection has a basis to favor genes that promote postreproductive longevity."

Nowadays, it is not the physical survival of the species that we are called upon to tend to, but postmenopausal wisdom is urgently needed for other purposes. Psychologist James Hillman has a particularly colorful way of describing the kind of fertility postmenopausal women have to offer: they may be "void of ova," he acknowledges in his book *The Force of Character,* but they are "packed with memes. Memes are the cultural equivalent of genes." Our generation has learned plenty about the world in our fast-moving first adulthood, and we are primed to pass it on, along with the wisdom we are accumulating as fast as we are transmitting it. The message, as Angier puts it, is: "What distinguishes women from all other primates, then, isn't menopause but the long, robust life that women can lead after menopause."

Betty Friedan, ever the iconoclast, sees the energy our generation is capable of generating in Second Adulthood as an agent of social transformation. In *The Fountain of Age,* written when she was seventy-two, she enthuses, "We have barely even considered the possibilities in age for new kinds of loving intimacy, purposeful work and activity, learning and knowing, community and care. . . . For to see age as continued human development involves a revolutionary paradigm shift."

Life Happens

Feistiness and energy can take you a long way, but there are some realities that won't yield to a simple no!—people you love, a job you hate, an aging parent, a financial loss. Still, the frame of mind that simple word promotes can make all the difference when shit happens.

And it happens more and more as we get older. Some of us are hit by a cataclysmic event—getting fired, getting sick, getting divorced—or difficult adjustments—going back to school or work, sending our last child out into the world, moving from a home of many years. Then there are those for whom a seismic shift takes place incrementally. The episodes add up almost imperceptibly, without seeming to change the narrative. Until one day, as Jyoti realized, "I had been throwing my pebbles into the wrong pond." She grew up in the deep South, where "feelings were not talked about, and families lived with so much despair . . . where women trying to go to women's circles were being beaten and divorced and killed." She fled with her children to Texas, where she became a social worker, but still felt her life wasn't working. "I was so discouraged," she admits. At forty-five, she left everything behind—including her grown children who disapproved of her decision to follow her spiritual calling—and found her way to the spiritual community she now leads. "After all the bad stuff," she says, "I wanted to be authentic. I wanted to be real."

Even though my own shake-up began with one of life's most traumatic events—I was asked to step down as editor of the magazine I had edited for seven years—it didn't feel like more than a temporary bump in the road. OK, I thought, I'll become a writer instead. I had been an editor for thirty years—seventeen of them in the exhilarating community of *Ms.* magazine. What I didn't understand then is that, although the elements—words—are the same for an editor and a writer, the practice is diametrically opposite. The difference lies in whose words they are. Running a magazine is primarily reactive—issuing assignments and decisions in response to the needs of the publication and the staff, making other people's words work, and talking, talking, talking. Writing is internal: pushing the brain to find new questions and to answer them in compelling ways. And any conversation that takes place is inside your own head. It is profoundly assertive, aggressive work, more active than anything I had done before. Although the material is still language, what shapes the words is my own message, what I think. The *no* voice has found much more to say. And it speaks the truth of what *I* know, regardless of what I have been told.

The voice that emerges in each of us in Second Adulthood can speak its mind to anything that life presents: a major financial decision, a deteriorating marriage, a health crisis, or a growing sense that it is time for a change.

BETTY'S STORY
"That Year Changed Me, Because I Became So Assertive"

Betty's is a particularly dramatic version of the *story of no*. A "life-altering event" made her realize at fifty-two that her life had, like many women I talked to, become "too narrow—or maybe had just stayed too narrow." She found that she was capable of much more.

Her first-adulthood choices were "traditional," perhaps because her childhood wasn't. "My mother had been a working mother"—both parents ran a family business—"when nobody else's mother was a working mother. And I hated it. I always wanted her home. I always felt the lack of her presence. . . . I could reach her by phone, but I rarely remember calling her. Now that I think of it, it was rare that I would talk to my Mom, and it wasn't for pleasure—only if there was some business or some crisis."

When Betty married, she "wanted to be a teacher of young children, then have babies and stay home." Which is what she did. By then, however, other women were exploring careers, and she felt "guilty and déclassé. But I couldn't help it. I wanted to be home. And I knew I was good at being a Mom."

She was less confident about being good at being wife. Her husband talked about divorce, and they went into therapy together. "I think I was not as interesting and stimulating as he thought I should be, as the working women who most of our friends were." The therapist said Betty was depressed and had low self-esteem. Over time the marriage recovered, but she continued to feel put down by the carefully phrased question "are you working outside the home?"

When her son David left for college and her daughter was in high school, Betty went back to teaching—and loved it. "I loved the teachers at my school, I loved my kids, I loved my principal! I loved the parents. They loved me. I was very happy!" She also felt more respect from her husband. As she entered her fifties, everything was falling into place. Here's how she describes what happened next:

"We were in this wonderfully relaxing small town on Lake Michigan, having a delightful, restful vacation, and then we were going to take off for Chicago, visit some relatives and go to the theater . . . Our son David was traveling in the Middle East with some friends, before starting a wonderful new job. While he was in Syria, unbeknownst to him, he got salmonella poisoning. And by the time he got to Israel—thank God he got to Israel when this happened—he began to feel terrible. He said to the friend he was with, 'You gotta get me to a hospital, I can't walk, I can't pick up this glass.' His friend and another friend got him to a hospital—by this time he really couldn't walk—and he was put into an ICU immediately.

"As we're packing up to set out for Chicago, we get the call every mother dreads: his friend saying he's in the emergency room. He hadn't been diagnosed yet, but they think he's dehydrated, so he'll probably be on the next plane home. We went back home to wait, and then we got the call saying it was Guillain-Barré syndrome. We didn't know what that was, but our first question was 'Should we come?' And the answer was 'No, he's probably going to be out in a couple of days.' But still we made all arrangements at that point, and we had a flight set up . . . and we got the next call that said 'Come, come now.'"

When Betty and her husband got there, David was on a ventilator. Two months later, still not breathing on his own, he was flown to a specialized hospital in Boston with Betty at his side. There she remained throughout his hospital stay and then at a rehab facility and finally at a wheelchair-accessible apartment building. A year in all. "That year changed me tremendously," she says, "because I became so assertive."

She became a shrewd and outspoken advocate for her beloved patient, who was a prisoner of the medical establishment. In Israel she quickly came to understand that she was considered in the way. "The role of mother was revered, provided it was restricted to holding her son's hand during visiting hours. But to want medical information, to want to be involved in the treatment, to get angry at the damn X-ray technician who wasn't holding David's head carefully . . . This was not very popular."

That was when she began to develop what she calls her "act." It "incorporated my whole basic personality of being very sweet and very ingratiating and deferential with a new 'OK, but now you will do as I say' kind of attitude."

Circumstances had pushed her headlong into the Fuck You Fifties, and, despite the tragic nature of the situation, she was glad to be there. "I felt so powerful. I had had no idea how powerful I could be! And it was a shocker. I had to do pretty much everything independently. I consulted with my husband on the phone, but there were so many decisions that I just had to make. I was living independently for the first time in my life. I had gone directly from college to an apartment my parents were paying for; and then I got married and, even though I was working, I was still being taken care of, still the old-fashioned wife. It had never been like this! I'd never lived on my own. And I was dealing with things that I would never have thought I could just do by myself."

After David left the hospital in April, Betty lived in the apartment with him until the end of August. "And then," she says, "he wanted me to go home. By then he had met the woman who he's now marrying. She was his speech therapist in the hospital. So I knew that he had someone, that if he needed something, she would come over, and so I left. And then I went back to my life."

But her life as she had led it up until the year before wasn't there for her to go back to. She hadn't lived full time with her husband for all those months; she hadn't been in touch with her friends and family. (In fact, her father had died during that year; the only time she left David alone for the night was to attend her father's funeral.) She couldn't imagine caring for anyone right then, even the preschoolers she loved teaching; and she was much tougher and self-sufficient than she had ever been before.

In that year, she had crossed into another state of mind. Today, she is not who she had been, only older. She has new skills, new confidence, and new priorities. So far, she has only a vague sense of what challenges she wants to take on. "Now my problem is, what direction am I going to go?" She isn't ready to step up to major life decisions yet, but she has made a crucial first commitment. She has said yes to herself. To Betty.

Growing up, her name had been Elizabeth Fran, and she shortened it to Betty. Then "around the time my husband was getting dissatisfied with me, and I was feeling dissatisfied with me, I started to wish I had kept Elizabeth. It sounded more imposing. When I started teaching, I used Elizabeth." But something happened during that year in Boston. "I started to feel more like Betty again. I felt I had abandoned my self when I went to Elizabeth. I realized that I didn't have to abandon the person who I really was to be a stronger version of that person, to be a more self-confident person. So I went back to Betty." That's the name she is using on the invitations to David's wedding—after which she looks forward to taking charge of her Second Adulthood.

———

Like Betty, none of us will know where we are going until we get there. But the adventure begins the first time we hear ourselves say no—loud and clear—to some version of what just doesn't feel right. As the no-longer-relevant, the never-authentic, and the overly-cautious is banished—one no! at a time—a source of energy and self-confidence is released that is sorely needed for the sorting-out process. For many of us, that means a year-or-two sojourn in an emotional free-fall zone—the Fertile Void—where we explore our options as though all bets are off.

CHAPTER FOUR

The Fertile Void

Taking Your Time

One day you finally knew
what you had to do, and began,
though the voices around you
kept shouting
their bad advice—
though the whole house
began to tremble
and you felt the old tug
at your ankles.
"Mend my life!"
each voice cried.
But you didn't stop . . .
. . . as you left their voices behind,
the stars began to burn
through the sheets of clouds,
and there was a new voice
which you slowly
recognized as your own,
that kept you company
as you strode deeper and deeper
into the world.
determined to do
the only thing you could do—
determined to save
the only life you could save.

—Mary Oliver, "The Journey"

Every woman I spoke to got the phrase "Fertile Void" the moment the words were out of my mouth. It didn't matter whether she had just been fired or promoted or whether she had been divorced or retired or had not changed her routine one bit, sooner or later each had found herself in a prolonged state of confusion just when she felt impelled to take action. They all felt the energy and spirit of adventure stirring, without knowing what kind of action to take.

Alexis is typical. She retired eighteen months ago from a long career as a high school teacher and coach of girls' sports, and she is still searching for her next commitment. "It's like this whole year has gone by and, in terms of things I thought I was going to get done, I think I've cleaned *one* kitchen drawer."

Rita is typical too. She has been in the same marriage and the same job and the same community for the past twenty years. She is beginning to sense winds of change but isn't ready to harness them yet. "I'm feeling that something is going to happen," she says, "but I think I'll be where I am for one more year."

Madeline is also typical. She is painfully extricating herself from a job of twenty-five years. "I knew it was time to go when I heard myself respond to a suggestion by saying, 'You can't do that. It won't work. We already tried it.'" She feels she has to move out of her first adulthood before she can make herself available to her second, but she longs to hear herself say, "I've *never* tried that; it might work." Whatever "that" might be.

Alexis and Rita and Madeline are all wondering what they are going to do with the rest of their lives. What makes Second Adulthood historic is that the question is coming up for midlife women at all. We know what "middle age" used to be about: cutting back, scaling down, giving up. And we know that isn't for us. At the same time we sense that doors are closing, that a chapter is over. We are no longer fertile; we are no longer the trend-setting generation; and we are now less likely to make a major mark. So we are torn between those "facts of life" and what we fear are "unrealistic expectations." Can I really learn a new language? Can I really start my own business? Can I fall in love? Get a divorce? Close up the house? Do I have what it takes to make changes in my life?

We are restless and curious and ready to get to work. The doubts and the "zest" create crosscurrents that can cancel each other out and leave us stymied by a sense of aimlessness. That is the Fertile Void. Traveling through it is an existential mission without a goal. Having goals at the start will only throw you off course. Meaningful goals will emerge in their own good time. But the unremitting unknowingness is hard to take.

"Anxiety is a rehearsal of the future," observed Gestalt therapy founder Fritz Perls, whose lectures are collected in *Gestalt Therapy Verbatim*. That panicky scramble to control the outcome of events that appear to be spinning out of control accompanies all the changes that characterize and destabilize Second Adulthood, from hormonal upheaval, to insecurity about finances, to fear of death. "This 'I don't know where I am' state creates anxiety for most people, because it is unknown territory," writes Ilana Rubenfeld, a student of Perls's, who coined the phrase "fertile void" to describe a crucial step in the process of change. "It is a time when your old ways do not work and you don't [yet] have new ways of coping."

The antidote to the anxiety of trying to get a grip on the future is, in Perls's view, to concentrate on the present, "the here-and-now." His advice is hard to apply to those crises when the future is literally at stake and solutions must be found to such practical problems as getting a job or paying unexpected bills. And some kinds of anxiety may also require medication or therapy. But the unknown territory of the Fertile Void is much more about the present than it may seem, and the anxiety over drifting there can be relieved just by not struggling to figure out what's next. While The Question—*What am I going to do with the rest of my life?*—dominates Second Adulthood, the journey toward it begins with a more existential inquiry: Who am I *now*?

The Fertile Void is a necessary, albeit bewildering, hiatus. Paradoxically, as Rubenfeld observed in her book *The Listening Hand,* it is "a place of change in which one sometimes feels 'stuck.'" For a proactive woman, the response to being "stuck" is to expend more energy, make more lists, go to more seminars, try to muster more will power, make more decisions. But the result, she often finds, is just spinning her wheels. The solution, ironically, is not more movement, but less. The cure for "stuck" is "still." A gathering in of the energy unleashed by Saying No and Letting Go. That is what the Fertile Void can offer, an opportunity to exchange the wish to control life for a willingness to engage living.

Of course, we are impatient. Up to now we have pushed through one stage after another—the adolescent wanting to be a woman, the woman wanting to be a wife, the mother wanting her kids to get just a little older so she could get some of her life back—hoping for something better. Looking ahead from here, however, we see very little to go on. That is because *ahead* is right now. The next stage is the shapeless process of the Fertile Void. "It is tempting to push through this stage quickly, to deny the struggles, fears and doubts," warns Rubenfeld. But, she adds, "by experiencing it fully, you will be able to continue on." In the zero gravity of the Fertile Void, The Question hits home.

Time Tyranny

One trouble is that "quickly" is our middle name. We have paced ourselves by the ethic of keeping up and speeding up and moving up, getting more done, doing *something,* not wasting time. Rubenfeld's reminder not to rush is almost an insult to the multitasking skills we have acquired at great expense during our adult lives. (I will never forget the working mother of three who epitomized the split-second timing her contemporaries perfected; "If I can shave both legs on the same day," she said, "I'm doing pretty well.")

Even if our present circumstances require that we keep up the pace, most of us have begun to feel uncomfortable in overdrive; simple burnout can make us want to slow to a walk. And the *mellowness*—the decreasing willingness to sweat the small stuff—that our changing brains lead us toward can make the flowers alongside the path smell very sweet. But there is no on/off switch to the pace. It takes time to break free of time.

The Fertile Void is where we make the transition from that driven, overcommitted superwoman to someone whose priorities and passions are less rigidly managed and perhaps more deeply felt. Stephen Covey, whose expertise is efficiency and effectiveness, makes an important distinction between what is "urgent" and what is "important." We can think of our first adulthood as driven by urgency, and our second as driven by importance.

A recently retired teacher describes this transition as a "kind of detox" from living by the bells that tolled her existence for thirty-five years. "I laughed about it, but in some ways I needed a bell to go to the bathroom. Everything was so structured." Yet she understands that while the limbo she is in "might look like no structure, it is not really no structure; it's really a *re*structuring. It takes time to decide what stays, what goes, what do I really need in my life?"

Most women report spending a year or more in the free fall from first adulthood into second. I spent two years there. After losing my job in a power struggle with my boss, I felt like a conductor without an orchestra. I installed a lovely new rolltop desk with lots of cubicles and drawers in the corner of my bedroom and took on freelance projects. I would sit at my computer and bang out things, interrupted by telemarketing calls and distracted by dust balls and unanswered mail. But deprived of the energizing uplift of being part of a familiar working group and deprived of being part of the drama of the news, I found that my day seemed unreal. *I* seemed unreal. In a kind of suspended animation. Without the defining structure of an office and colleagues, I didn't feel like a grown-up. The upside was that I saw more of my two teenage kids and became more in tune with the rhythm of their days. The downside was that I became more intrusive in their lives. I brought little to the end-of-day conversations with my husband and less income to the family. Over the years I had gone to an office, my apartment had become my housekeeper's daytime domain. When I was there, too, I felt like an intruder in my own environment and a lost soul in everyone else's.

I kept asking myself The Question: what's next? There was no reply. People tried to be helpful by posing other questions: "Do you want to take a full time job?" "Do you want to go back to school?" "How about writing annual reports?" "Do you want to retire?" "Didn't you always want to paint?" None of which were helpful, because I simply wasn't ready to answer them. I needed more time. I needed time to make peace with time.

For me, as for most women, time had become an enemy,

an unappeasable tyrant. I had become a master of time management—I would warm food in the microwave at either 1 minute, 2–3 seconds or 2 minutes, 3–4 seconds because it was faster to push adjoining buttons—but there were always short-cuts I hadn't thought of. I once met a woman who dressed her children before they went to bed to save time in the morning. Getting things done had been my highest—my only—priority. I would choose an errand over a trip to the bathroom. I would stop having fun way before I needed to because I was anticipating upcoming demands. I was overbooked but determined to prove (to whom? I now wonder) that I could "manage."

"Hurry sickness" is the name James Gleick gives, in his book *Faster,* to the modern epidemic of time-tyranny. He quotes an expert in "biological time" who cites jet lag as the quintessential example of what it feels like to impose external time on internal time: "that disconcerting sensation of time travelers that their organs are strewn across a dozen time zones while their empty skins still forge boldly into the future." That sounds like the kind of time-bind most of the women I know can experience on an average day!

When I no longer had to live on a schedule that put me at the mercy of my watch, I felt like I was swimming through a miasma of undifferentiated hours and minutes. On days when I had three things to do, I would panic that I wouldn't get them done; and when there was nothing I had to do on a particular day, I would lie in bed and wait for something to happen.

Little by little, I began to rebuild my relationship with time. I took added delight in lunch with a friend when I didn't have to check whether we had been there over an hour. I realized that I had stopped reading for pleasure, because I hated doing it in short, stolen or interrupted doses. I was in heaven now that I could settle in for a hundred pages at a time. I found that work didn't need to take place only in daylight hours, that early morning or late night sometimes felt right. I discovered that cooking wasn't a chore, if the planning, shopping, and preparing didn't have to be orchestrated like the invasion of Normandy, but could, in fact, be done in a satisfying sequence on the same day. Even though I am still plagued by residual hurry sickness—when putting on sneakers and socks, I brood about which is more efficient, sock-sock-sneaker-sneaker or sock-sneaker-sock-sneaker—I am better able to take *my* time. And I am gaining clarity about what I want to do with it.

Judy, a successful executive who became a consultant a few years ago, is experiencing the Fertile Void as an effort to stop speeding past life itself. "I spent so much of my life rushing that I am now trying to slow down enough to experience the texture of life." She devotes much of her time to her aging parents. Last year, she joined her 90-year-old father on a business trip to China, and she is "orchestrating the care" of her mother who has Alzheimer's. As Judy is quick to point out, experiencing "the texture of life" is not a leisure activity. "A lot of it is hard," she admits. And disruptive. Resetting her own pace put Judy in a different time zone from her husband. While she was free to spend weeks at a time in the Maine cabin she and her husband have lovingly restored over the last twenty years, her absence left him feeling rejected and resentful. The discrepancy between her textured time frame and his nine-to-five schedule led to some soul-searching about the marriage, and recently her husband decided to go back to school—in Maine. Ironically, he is more excited than she is about leaving the city behind.

Judy is adjusting to the difference between the unrelenting tick of the clock that has ruled her life for so long and the rhythmic beat of a human heart that speeds up and slows down according to what is being experienced. As long as we live by the maxim that time is money, we forget that time is life. We need to become attuned to other rhythmic measures of our days. Many religions find inspiration in the rhythmic heartbeat of ceremonial drums. They understand, writes Dr. Stephan Rechtschaffen, founder of the Omega Institute for Holistic Studies and author of *Timeshifting,* "the power of rhythm to transform mundane or profane time into sacred time, where contemplation supersedes pace, where timelessness overcomes social time." Ideally, that is what takes place in the Fertile Void.

Getting to What's Next

The further we get into renegotiating our relationship with time, the closer we get to the ultimate power of time—to run out. Karen Van Allen, who is a psychotherapist, got there about six years ago. She realized that between the time she was a teenager who believed she would live forever and recent years when she has begun to face the fact that she won't, she hadn't thought much about her mortality. She began to see that facing what is lost with age is the first step toward finding the passions that will fire the discoveries that await us before time runs out.

Together with Ruth Neubauer, another psychotherapist who had come to the same place in her own life, Karen has devised a weekend program and six-week discussion groups for women over fifty. It's called "Retirement or What Next." Here is how their brochure describes the objectives of the twice-yearly workshops:

To meet the needs of women (50+) who through *external events* (retirement, divorce, "empty nest," death of parents, ill-

ness of a spouse . . .) or *internal pressures* (restlessness, long-
ings, uncertainty, feeling overloaded . . .) realize that a change
is needed, but to what is unknown. If you feel pressure to
respond to the question "What do I do with the rest of my
life?" . . . know what you want to do but feel inhibited . . .
wish to express yourself in new ways . . . want support to play
with ideas and dreams . . . plan to retire and have concerns.

Their experience over the past several years with nearly one
hundred women, in groups of ten or twelve, who have gathered to share their confusion and find their way, has given the
two therapists some insights into the nature of the Fertile Void,
which they laid out for me.

Their first general observation is counterintuitive to the expectations we have for ourselves, but confirms what we are beginning to understand about Second Adulthood. "It's been
fascinating," says Ruth, "And unexpected." No matter how di-
vergent the life stories are—" 'I've never had children,' or 'I'm
in a long-term marriage,' or 'I've been divorced twice,' or 'my
husband just left,' or 'I've always had a job,' or 'I've never had a
job'"—the question is the same. Every woman who has been
attracted to the program is there because, says Ruth, she knows
"It's time for me to look at what I'm doing with my life, and
what I really care about is that it has some meaning for me." She
is there to meet her true self.

Their second observation is about how hard it is to get the
women in their groups to downshift into what Ruth calls *real*
time. "We try to slow them down, so that for two days there
isn't anything external. It is structured—we start on time and
we end on time—but within that there is a lot of freedom and,
we hope, a chance to experience having your internal and external lives in sync."

As we explored the notion of integrating the personal and performance pieces of our lives, I thought of all the women I had met for whom that reunification is the real quest of Second Adulthood. Like a repertory actor, a fifty-year-old woman has played so many roles and found herself in so many different dramas and comedies over the season of her adult life, that when it is time to move on, she finds herself on the empty stage costumed in the equivalent of a medieval wimple on her head, a Brechtian shawl around her shoulders, a Joan of Arc breastplate, *Chorus Line* fishnet stocking on one leg, and an assembly line work boot on the other. The accumulated accessories no longer enhance the actor underneath; they obscure her. She wants to pack all that away—and get back to reality. Whether you call it "self" or "authenticity" or "identity" or "integrity" or "taking responsibility for your life," you simply can't leave home—the home of our lives so far—without it.

Unlike many other programs that promise to help women make transition decisions, "Retirement or What Next" is designed to *explore* the Fertile Void, not just get through it. The exercises Ruth and Karen offer their groups are helpful. Together we extrapolated some guidelines.

Get to Know The Question. "What am I going to do with the rest of my life? is not a light question," says Ruth, "and there is no to-do answer. In the group we try to hold onto the question and allow for the messiness of not knowing the answer." The Question just sits there for as long as it takes. As each woman reframes the question in the context of her own experience, the others come to appreciate the gravity of the inquiry. If anyone starts to offer advice—to *fix* whatever is broken—Ruth and Karen shift the conversation away from what they call the *I'll take care of you* track. "When someone starts saying, 'Well, what you should do is to get your husband to nananana . . .' you can see the other woman shrivel," says Karen. "You know how it is when someone is giving you advice you don't want? You just shrivel."

When anxiety or impatience creeps in, Ruth and Karen reassure the women that they know from experience that each one has the answer or *an* answer she needs. "You might not know what it is," Karen tells them. "You might not know what it is by the end of our weekend or even six months from now, but something is there, and at the end of this weekend you are going to be somewhere you can identify on this journey. You are going to have moved. You'll have different questions to ask yourself."

Again, the bottom line is: it takes time. The rhythm-of-life kind, not the tick-tock kind. Ruth recalled a "perky, funky" woman who had struggled in the group with a growing feeling of discomfort from what she felt were arbitrary limitations being imposed on her. She couldn't identify the source of her claustrophobia and she couldn't imagine how to break free. A year later she called Ruth out of the blue and left a "perky, funky little message" on the answering machine. "I just wanted to tell you," she said, "that I've left the job—no more rules, no more regs. And I bought the house! And I'm so happy."

Listen to Yourself. It isn't easy to sit still for yourself. Especially, Ruth points out, "when we're uncomfortable. And this is uncomfortable stuff, because there's something nagging, and you don't know what it is, and you don't know what to do about it, with a capital *do*." In the workshop Ruth and Karen try to provide an environment in which the women feel that nothing is expected of them. They can just stay uncomfortable, if that is where they are. "In the end, something comes together," adds Ruth, "even if it's just knowing you are unhappy with what you are doing."

Not having to do something is easier said than done. We live by to-do lists, and our first presumption about Second Adulthood is that it presents just one more list. So we dutifully line up an agenda of tasks. Typically, it calls for more than a few cleaning-out projects—the attic, the garage, the closets, the memories drawer. And then we don't do them. But if you pay attention to your state of mind, you can detect a profound impulse behind the mundane lists: to get rid of the detritus of the first adulthood and pack up What Matters for the journey to the next one. "You can't really move on until you have cleared out the clutter," says Ruth.

A woman who came to a *What Next?* weekend was very impatient with herself for not getting off her butt and cleaning out her basement. When she took the time to sit still with herself, however, she realized that what she was really telling herself was to get rid of the garbage in her life. That was a slightly bigger job. There is only one voice that counts when she confronts that garbage, one voice that has the power of the Queen of Hearts in *Alice in Wonderland* to pronounce, "Off with her head!" to this or that piece of flotsam. That is the voice being unmuffled in the Fertile Void.

Tune In to What Turns You On. "This is often very poignant," says Karen, "because a lot of women say, 'I don't know.' It is very frightening for them. They don't know if they care about anything."

Again the answer can only come from the unmuffled voice. "We have to make room for that small voice that says, 'I really don't know . . . but I think maybe . . . I used to . . .'" she urges. "A lot of us don't have big passions, like 'I knew from the time

I was three I was going to be a concert pianist,' so we have to issue an invitation to even a little flicker of interest." In the groups, the invitations Ruth and Karen have designed are meant to get beneath the to-do mind-set. They include playing music and encouraging the women to move to it, reading poetry, writing, drawing with bright colors, anything that will "turn off the censors," those nagging voices that tell us our dreams are silly or impractical or irresponsible. Or, worst of all, "selfish."

As they talked about passions, both therapists remembered one of their first clients. "She'd always had this dream," recalls Karen, "a very tiny dream, but a persistent one—of volunteering in an animal shelter. That's what she found on her plate. And she did it!"

Another woman, a financial expert all her life, expected that when she retired she would continue to work with individual clients. But she had always wanted to travel, too. In the course of a weekend, the travel wish began to, as Karen puts it, "pick up steam." It moved off the sidelines and met up with the "ascendant" idea of starting a small consulting business. Three years later, this woman takes groups of women on tours to out-of-the-way places, and her business card says *world traveler* along with *financial consultant.*

Stop Listening to Others. This step deals with another muffle on a woman's full voice. Ruth and Karen call it "breaking through injunctions. Whose voice is it in your head that says, 'This is not okay'? Who do you hear and what are they saying?" Most often the voice is a parent or a teacher, but it can be an older sibling, or anyone who has passed judgment on your self-expression. "There are a lot of obstacles in our way," says Ruth. "And the question is what are they? And who says they are there? And what if you pretended they weren't there?"

In place of the naysayers, Ruth and Karen suggest imagining a "personal board of directors" composed of people you know or people you don't know—"the Dalai Lama if you want," or a character from literature or the movies—who are "on your side." Picture them sitting there listening, taking you seriously, and offering encouragement; it makes it easier to imagine firing those who are not on your side. The objective is not to turn to outside "experts" for solutions but to establish new voices in your own internal dialogue. As one woman put it, "I found myself saying things I knew all along—but 'didn't know' until then."

Speaking up for yourself involves making choices on your own say-so. The choices may not be ideal, but they are your choices—formed from the yin-yang of Letting Go and Saying No. "Once you feel it's okay to make choices, without feeling guilty or listening to the voice that says 'you should be doing this or that,'" says Ruth, "then the loss of a choice—the road not taken—is much less painful."

Letting Go. "We talk a lot about loss, and grieving, and ritual, and leaving time for that, for saying goodbye," says Ruth. There are moments when it may seem as if nothing will be left once the leftovers and false prophets of a lifetime are cleaned out. And there are moments when the old ways start to look awfully good. "For every opening of a new idea or just seeing the light come in in a new way, means you are letting go of something, and that doesn't feel good. Even," she adds, "if what you are letting go of hasn't been good."

"Part of our time together is about grief. We're quite explicitly reassuring here. 'You will be okay. There will be something there,'" adds Ruth. "We had one woman," recalled Karen, "who came in and just started crying. She was fine but that was exactly what she needed to do. She needed to be with her feelings of loss and accept what she was going through. She was quite fine at the end."

A common sense of loss has to do with physical appearance and capability. Every woman in every group bemoans memory lapses or reading glasses or lost waistlines. But some were relieved to let go of the constant preoccupation with looks. One woman finally said goodbye to the assumption—a bond between her mother, her sisters, and herself—that a woman has to make keeping up her appearance a top priority to "keep a man." She realized, to her surprise and delight, that if she cut back on manicures, shopping expeditions, and regular waxings and facials, she would have more time and energy to devote to the other things she now realized she wanted to get to.

The "letting go" step of the workshop also concentrates on shedding the shoulda-woulda-coulda thinking around past life choices. "Whether you had children, or didn't; whether you married the person you should have; all of those things come under the category of things that need to be relinquished, in order to get on with the rest," says Karen. Paradoxically, the same applies to future choices. Karen recalled a woman who had developed a clear game plan for her retirement. "She knew exactly what she was going to do. She had set the date, she had managed the money. Then her husband got terribly ill, and she had to become his full-time caregiver. There are so many examples of best laid plans going awry: 'I thought I was going to do this and then I got arthritis or breast cancer or my husband left me . . .' You can't be too attached to ideas. Even if you figure everything out, you can't get too attached to it."

In place of the best-laid plans, we are building a new

resource—a mellow confidence in our ability to cope with and even embrace what life brings. So while we cannot let go of the grief and fear that come with a heightened awareness of mortality, we can let go of the notion that we can do anything about it. It frees up psychic energy to stop trying to get a grip on "things that we can't control in the first place," says Ruth. Letting go of the illusion of control is so hard for most of us, but it opens up the way to new solutions. A friend whose husband is very ill told me she confided to her therapist that she wanted to "either cure him or kill him." To which the therapist replied dryly, "well, since you can't do either, let's explore some other options."

At the end of one weekend something happened that, when Ruth described it, gave me a mental image for the amorphous Fertile Void experience. As members of the group were saying goodbye to each other, one woman wandered out into Ruth's garden and stood at the trellis archway leading into the surrounding woods. It was as though she was literally stuck to the ground. Then, as if gathering strength from the stillness, she strode briskly through the arch and into the woods, turned around, and came right back. "I had so much trouble walking out of your garden into the woods. I felt I was walking out on my old life," she told Ruth. "But finally I did it. And coming back was much easier." For one thing she had left behind some of the baggage she had arrived with, so she was traveling light; but most important, she was now traveling on her own psychic steam, by her own choice. And, to her amazement, she had not become a stranger in a strange land—she was moving on with her life, not walking out on it. "When I came back I saw the garden in a completely different way," she told Ruth. When I pictured this moment, I was reminded of Vivi's poignant discovery of her "desert eyes" that enabled her to see the vitality in superficially barren terrain. A sojourn in the Fertile Void doesn't necessarily change our circumstances, but it does change the way our lives look to us.

When they go back home, the women who take the Retirement or What Next workshop still have questions, but not the ones they came in with. Ruth suggests some of the new versions: "How do I get my life lined up so I'm living it?" or "How can I live in a way that says this is who I am?" Then she zeroes in on the Second Adulthood theme of integrating and asserting one's self. "I think what isn't getting talked about," says Ruth, "is the inauthentic and the authentic, or the external and the internal, and where the disconnect is. What is happening is that the women who come to our groups want to be connected to *themselves*."

In the Gnostic Gospels (teachings of Jesus recorded within a century of his death and only discovered in recent years), Jesus is reported to have said "If you bring forth what is within you, what you bring forth will save you. If you do not bring forth what is within you, what you do not bring forth will destroy you." The Fertile Void is where the choice is made.

ALEXIS'S STORY
"I Had Been Feeling That I Was Pissing Away the Time . . ."

As crucial as it is, the Fertile Void can feel like wasted time or an aimless interlude until you are on the other side of it. Alexis now sees her first two years of retirement as "a quest," but at the time her random actions didn't seem to add up. As someone who was "always running around like a chicken with her head cut off"—on the high school coaching staff, raising her kids, rolling with the tides of a thirty-year marriage, being active in political organizations, square dancing, playing tennis and golf—the change of pace was disconcerting, to say the least.

It isn't in her nature to let life happen to her. She had always been a step-up-to-the-plate kind of person. Back when she was a young teacher and coaching girls' basketball, she defied the school administration and ended up in court for seven years. "There was this big ball game and they needed the girls' locker room to bring the boys team in," she explained to me. "We had something like thirty-four lockers and about one hundred fifty girls sharing them. So I said, 'No, I'm not asking the girls to move their things out of their locker room. You can use one of the other eleven locker rooms in the building.' But ours was the closest and the newest—Title IX was just beginning to take effect"—banning sex discrimination in school programs. "I don't know what the rationale was other than they just wanted to disrupt us. The upshot was they went into our locker room, broke open all the lockers, took out all the girls stuff and threw it into an office space. Over $500 worth of private property was lost or destroyed. It was pretty gruesome." Another upshot was that Alexis was fired for insubordination.

"So what did you do next?" I asked. "I kept teaching," she explained. "I was only fired from the coaching job." The court case went up to the state supreme court before being thrown out on a technicality. Alexis went to work every day among her adversaries. "It was just horrible," she says. "But I'm like a billy goat; I'm stubborn that way. It's just part of my personality. And of course I needed the job. In the end, though, I outlasted them—they all have died or retired—and I think I set a standard. I was in a position of helping young people work through some new jobs and things like that, and they would often say,

'But we're not like you,' and I would say, 'yes, you are.' I think I moved to a position where you don't mess with me!'"

After retiring at fifty-three, her days became less dramatic and her style less insubordinate. She feels guilty about not being proactive in the don't-mess-with-me mode she became known for. Instead, she is filling the Fertile Void with activities and people that instinct tells her will answer The Question. "I really enjoy golf and lots of my friends are golfing, so I get to be with them, and that's a good thing. I love the opera. I love theater. I play bridge—it was really exciting to be able to play bridge three times a week instead of once a month." When her husband was unexpectedly forced to retire, she was briefly thrown off her game. "I was angry at first," she admits; "this was supposed to be my time for myself." But they began doing small home-improvement jobs around the house and "kind of trying to refocus what we like to do together." And she manages to see more of her ten siblings and stay in touch with the young teachers she has mentored, as well as with her children and grandchildren. When she considers those young people, she wants to "set an example for them . . . by doing what I want to do, by being the best in these things that I love." Whatever they may be.

When she tried to describe to her daughter how guilty she felt about squandering her retirement, her daughter reassured her. "'Mom' she said. 'You're a kid in a candy story. It's like suddenly you have this time and you can say, 'yes, I can do that, sure I can do that . . .' and it's all great fun.'" But Alexis still felt she needed to "get organized." Then one day she was reviewing her retirement so far with her sister, and a pattern began to emerge. It was as though the interests floating around the boundaries of her life suddenly met Velcro at the center. What she *didn't* want to do was build up more accomplishments or focus on one thing; what she really *wanted* to do right now was pay attention to all aspects of her life, to experience the whole of who she is.

"I was going through some of the things that I enjoyed doing during my retirement," she recalls, "and my sister says, 'Well, let's see what's going on. You've got your physical self, and your intellectual self, and there's your social self, and then'—she's a real Bible Thumper—'you don't want to forget your spiritual self.' And she says, 'How are we going to remember that; we need an acronym: P for physical, I for intellectual, S for social, and S for spiritual, you have . . .' "

Alexis laughed at the recollection of their simultaneous hilarity. "I had been feeling that I had been 'pissing' away the time . . . But now that I have this acronym, I can get to work on really PISSing. I have a focus now." The focus is that unique mix of emotions and experiences and relationships that Alexis is now reweaving into a Second Adulthood identity that is not who she was, only older. That identity may resemble the responsible, organized, and effective personna of her first adulthood, or it may be a variation on other themes. Her Fertile Void mission, if she had been conscious of it, was to identify the pieces of her true self she wanted to carry forward. Her goal now is to assemble them into an updated identity. That, she will find, involves reassembling the elements of her life, as well, and recalibrating her commitments to work, family, friends, community, and her own passions. She will find that those months in the Fertile Void were not lost but a necessary preparation.

———

The great and innovative psychoanalyst Erik Erikson spent a lifetime studying and (beginning in 1959) writing about identity and the life cycle, but it was his wife and co-author, Joan, who wrote the final chapter, the one that speaks to us now. By then she had passed through her own Second Adulthood. The Eriksonian model of development establishes a pair of affirming and destructive challenges to psychological growth at every life stage. In this scheme, during the stage I call first adulthood (and Erikson calls *adulthood*) we are consumed by the need to make a mark and haunted by the fear of incompetence and irrelevance. But those preoccupations dissipate in the next stage and give way to the twin forces of *integrity* and *despair.* Despair is characterized by cynicism, dogmatism, and pessimism—qualities we all recognize from our bad days. It is with the alternative notion of Integrity that Joan Erikson, who continued writing about their work after her husband's death, speaks to Alexis and to the women in Ruth and Karen's group. Integrity, she writes in an introduction to *The Life Cycle Completed,* "is a wonderfully challenging word. It demands no strenuous deliberation or performance, just everyday management of all major and minor activities, with all the steadfast attention to detail necessary for a day well lived. It is all so simple, so direct, and *so difficult.*"

The Fertile Void is the long, slow, deep breath—the gathering in of strength—that precedes a daring leap into the unknown. Teetering on the brink is the stuff nightmares are made of, yet taken in slow motion, the same loss of balance becomes more dreamlike. The Fertile Void can be where we let go of demons and demands we don't need anymore and begin building new dreams, one well-lived day at a time.

Finding Out What Works: Recalibrating Your Life

CHAPTER FIVE

Reconsidering Work and Beginning to Recalibrate Your Life

Self-development is a higher duty than self-sacrifice. The thing which most retards and militates against women's self-development is self-sacrifice.

—Elizabeth Cady Stanton, suffragist, 1848

Nearly twenty-two million women over forty-five are in the workforce. According to the Bureau of Labor Statistics, the number of women over fifty-five who are employed will grow more than 50 percent by 2010—despite the rampant ageism in our culture. So pervasive is the expectation of earning a living in our generation that when we begin to ask ourselves The Question, we usually frame it in terms of work—going back to it, retiring from it, changing it, changing its hours. And we attribute the queasiness we experience at the edge of the Fertile Void to anxiety about implementing the work decision—a decision that will, we hope, materialize any minute. As the journey continues, and a game plan remains elusive, it becomes clear that we are questioning much more, *including,* but not only, the place we want—and need—to hold work in our lives. The problem is: the outlook from the Fertile Void is boundless and maddeningly amorphous, but when we focus on work, the prospect is circumscribed and deadly practical. Many of the considerations, financial and otherwise, are intractable, and the obstacles are real.

To complicate things even further, many of the expectations we have about work are more emotional than rational. For our generation, working embodies the transformation of women's experience that took place during our first adulthood. Back when many of us started working—in the seventies—a paycheck of one's own assumed magical powers beyond the daily grind that going to work usually is. A job "outside the home" signified self-sufficiency, taking adult control of our lives, and an opportunity for self-discovery. Getting paid for one's contribution to society commanded authority and respect. Even women who chose to become fulltime homemakers found work to be a defining factor. Just when they made their decision to stay home—some time in the 1980s—the balance shifted. Those who didn't regret their choice often still felt left behind; many of them are hoping to get into the game now. Working enabled thousands of women to find their talents and to experience power, to leave bad marriages and to support their children—to live as they chose. No wonder the prospect of reconsidering its place in our lives is anxiety-producing.

Making a decision about work is often the first of many adjustments a woman will undertake to recalibrate her life in the course of her Second Adulthood journey. If, as experience confirms, you are not who you were, only older, then before taking action in any arena, you have to ask yourself how your shifting priorities have changed the landscape. The Question, as it pertains to work prompts several levels of inquiry.

What matters? has changed dramatically for most of us since we first looked at the world of work. A recent survey of over 1,200 readers of *More*—a lifestyle magazine for women in their forties and fifties, three-quarters of whom are employed—found that "traveling (63 percent) and new hobbies (52 percent) are more important than career (35 percent) or volunteer work (29 percent)." (As further evidence of a major shift in priorities at this stage, "eating a healthy diet," "maintaining old friendships," and "having time for yourself" ranked above "spouse/significant other.")

For another segment of Second Adulthood women, myself included, work is still at the top of the list. It is where we find satisfaction, excitement, financial security, and, in part, escape from the personal and family questions that beset us. But even for us, priorities have changed. Ambition has given way to self-fulfillment; the need for recognition has been replaced by self-assurance, success by achievement, and knowing the ropes by learning new things.

In both groups, the focus has moved from outside in. From dependence on the environment to dependence on self. Each of us is trying to understand where work fits into the discoveries we are making about who we are now. Whether a woman is going to work for the first time, is being promoted to CEO, or is retiring, she is responding to a newly elevated Second Adulthood imperative: self-expression. That may mean finding a way of working at the speed and level that suits her, or under circumstances that allow her to be totally devoted to the work at hand. Or it may mean exploring new options—paid or unpaid—or new ways of working that engage her faculties, her imagination, her passion. It may even mean giving up work as she knows it for experiences that delight or captivate her mind, or making a commitment to a cause or a project or a person in a way that is reflective of her best self. As we consider work options—limited as they may be by economic and other practical factors—it is important to keep in mind that we are not the workers we were, only older.

The women I met are all trying to figure out what has changed, but each woman's insight is different. "I've gotten as far as I am going to get" is a common observation, but so is, "I'm just not as ambitious as I used to be. I'm kind of enjoying just doing what I do well." The objectives of money, recognition, independence, and self-expression have always been in the mix, but at different times in our lives one or another has taken precedence. Now that is about to happen again. Second Adulthood, we are beginning to see, is about reshuffling the whole deck.

Ellen realized too late that the reflex that had taken her from one professional challenge to the next all of her working life had propelled her right past an important choice. When her grandson was born, she was offered an opportunity to take over a large organization. By the time the dust of the new job had settled, her son and his family had moved across the country, and she had lost the option of daily contact with this child who was changing every day. "I think I made a real mistake," she admitted. Her priorities had shifted without her being aware of it.

For Sarah, on the other hand, who has been marking time at a midlevel job, her priorities were becoming crystal clear. "I want to put my ducks in order," she said, "so the minute my child needs me less, I can leap on something. It's nice to be interested in lots of things, but I don't want to be scattered. I want to be like a rocket ship that's going to go off!"

In Crystal's case, serendipity found her just as her last child went off to college. A chance encounter with a master potter who worked in the Cherokee tradition opened the door for Crystal, also a Native American, and her talent exploded. She was recently singled out as one of the Indian "artists to watch" after only five years of work. "We all have passions in our lives," she says. "When we reach a certain age, we should concentrate on pursuing those. For me it is a way to contribute to society, and it provides a sense of personal fulfillment."

To reconsider the work piece of our lives, we need to shed outdated assumptions about what we expect and need from the work we do and about what we are prepared to bring to it now. It's important for each of us—especially those who have had long-standing dreams about working, but haven't yet put them to the test—to seriously reevaluate What Matters in a job in terms of what matters to us *now.*

We Are Not the Workers We Were, Only Older

For many the defining ingredient in the work experience so far has been work–family tension. We became the trade-off generation, bartering time for money, life for sleep, and ambition for an approximation of balance. Among women who did not marry or have children, some feel they made the biggest trade-off of all, and they may want to recapture some bypassed life experiences in their Second Adulthood. For those who have walked the work tightrope, many of those demands will subside, and the working world is going to look very different.

As a result of that work–family push-pull, we have carved out an anomalous career path. The conventional (male) model of professional development is the *ladder*—geometric, if you will. Ours is more organic. Two management professors, Connie J. G. Gersick, director of the Institute for Leadership at Yale, and Kathy E. Kram at the Boston University School of Management, have identified what they call the "zig-zag" work pattern of women now in their late forties and fifties. Beginning with modest expectations—we were told to get a teaching certificate, just to be on the safe side—they got caught up in the work dynamic of the seventies and their expectations and satisfactions grew. Then came a plateau when family life and work were in conflict, and a woman had to run as fast as she could just to stay in place. Now, the study reports, the women they interviewed "describe a sense of coming into one's own, of newfound confidence in their abilities, of zest and new learning that they had not experienced." Employers may be skeptical of the zigzag, but it may serve us well as we move forward. After all, ladders go only so high, with room for only one at the top; zigs and zags can be endlessly innovative and resourceful and inclusive.

RITA'S STORY
"I Don't Care if I Had a Husband Who Kissed My Toes,
I Would Have Hated That Job!"

It is hard to disengage from assumptions, based on the zigzag experience, about how the demands of work and family will interact in the future—and where *life* fits in. Rita's story is an example of how inextricably intertwined these twin forces have been for so many women. She got married at twenty-one, while still in college, to a lawyer a few years older. Within a year she was pregnant. A miscarriage nearly derailed her, but a woman professor encouraged her to keep working at her thesis. She finished it—"seventy pages, and all in French!" It is still one of her most prized accomplishments. When she got pregnant and miscarried again, she was "devastated." What made it worth getting up each day was her new job, teaching French. "I have always loved languages," she says. "And I loved the teaching."

When her gynecological problems were solved, she quickly had three children. They became her top priority—and her great satisfaction. After a decade, when she was able to inch back to work part time, she created a course at a local community college for people traveling to Paris who wanted to learn French. "It was a wonderful class," she remembers. "I had presidents of banks, superintendents of schools, really neat people." Briefly her work (part time) and family (full time) were in balance. She was in what the zigzag study identifies as a "holding pattern."

When her youngest child entered school, she took a full-time job teaching in the local high school. "I hated it. You see 150 kids a day. Five classes and homeroom. They were like *Lord of the Flies.* It's torture. Especially if you are an intense person who wants to do the job well." About the same time, her marriage hit bottom when she discovered that her husband was having an affair. The therapist she consulted "thought my self-esteem problems were from my husband's affair," she says, but Rita understood that there was another factor in the equation. "I just hated my teaching job. I don't care if I had a husband who kissed my toes, I would have still hated that job!"

She and her husband worked things out, and she found a teaching position that she liked much better. With his help at home, she also went back to school—an hour's commute—to get certification to teach Spanish as well as French. Her sense of accomplishment was kicking in. "That was one of the best years of my life, even though I got a couple of speeding tickets getting from one piece of my life to another."

Today Rita teaches English as a Second Language in the local federal prison. It is the high point of her working life. "When you teach college in prison, they give up their blood—that's all they have—as opposed to kids, who suck your veins." For protection, she wears a body alarm but has never had to use it. "Some of the lessons I've had there have been incredible. I feel like I've become such a good teacher. The classes are three hours long, so you have to do so much. Sometimes I teach them songs, because I love music; I've talked about *West Side Story* and the song 'There's a Place for Us.' There are days when I feel there is someone over me, making everything work . . ."

Even so, Rita, who just turned fifty-five, is restless. With her children out in the world and her husband not anxious to retire, the coast is clear. She is beginning to reshuffle the pieces of her life. "It will be interesting to see what I'll do next, " she muses. One thing she looks forward to is a new stage of family life, becoming a grandmother—"that's my dream, if you want to know the truth"—but that isn't in the cards right now. As far as work goes, "I'd like to do something totally different." What had been her work—languages—may be recast as a hobby. "Did I tell you," she announced with delight at the end of our conversation, "I am starting to learn Chinese! I have a lot of Chinese inmates so I'm starting to pick it up. The problem is finding a class. I have a friend, a young woman from Beijing. She just got a piano, so I am going to teach her piano and she is going to teach me Chinese. . . ." Rita can see herself as a yoga instructor or perhaps in a horticulture business, but when she tries to imagine herself in a different work context, she realizes it will call upon qualities that she hadn't previously associated with work. "It might be hard for me to sit quietly and work with plants," she wonders. But it might *not* be so hard. The compartmentalized elements—job, family, hobbies, *me*—can interact in ways the worker we were in the past couldn't imagine.

Work as Caregiving—and Caregetting

Playing well with others has been almost a way of life since childhood. Many women have thrived in service jobs that take advantage of the interpersonal sensitivity neuroscientists call executive social skills and in which we excel. Careers in sales, law, teaching, and psychology have given thousands of women status and satisfaction in recent years. These same skills have brought women success in behind-the-scenes jobs. Every office has the motherly manager who always seems to know when something is wrong and drops everything to tend to it. Every company has the woman who makes sure the hot-tempered executives don't take the whole place down with them. There are countless women whose mission is not to let the team down. Because it has been a guiding principle for so many of us for so long, it is important to disengage from the "I like working with people" assumption—at least long enough to reconsider it.

The rewards of being able to tune into another person's needs—and sometimes to answer them—are many, as we know; but the cost to our own needs can be high. When the women I talked to reviewed what had been lacking in their first adult-hood, self-nurturing moved to the top of the list. How, then, do we reconfigure our days to answer to ourselves as attentively as we have answered to others? For some doing the work itself—because it is exciting, meaningful, or financially rewarding—is how we care for ourselves. For others detaching somewhat from the caregiving environment we have made of the workplace will set free a sense of new possibility similar to what we feel when demands of the primary caregiving commitment are lifted.

Of course, working with people has a crucial care*getting* component, as well. As sociologist Arlie Russell Hochschild observed in *The Time Bind,* given the lack of support for fam-ily life, many people feel their work life is more manageable and enriching than their home life. She was writing about the wrenching demands of raising children, but it seems equally true that when the house begins to empty out, the other fam-ily can look even more inviting. Nevertheless, that may no longer be the kind of relationship a particular woman craves from her work. She may want to seek community elsewhere. That was my experience.

As I moved from being part of a team to going solo, my thirty years of community was the hardest component to disengage from my notion of work. Throughout my first adulthood, I had counted on the support of a group of women I trusted. I remember, during a particularly rough patch in my marriage, a colleague and I formed what we called the Thank God It's Monday Club in recognition of how, after a weekend of self-doubt and conflict, we could take pride in the work we did together and, most important, we could *laugh* about it all.

When I left that tight-knit and nurturing community for freelance work, I tried to approximate it by taking office space in the midst of a friendly and compatible organization, but to my surprise I found myself craving privacy. The companionship quotient had shifted from casual crackling camaraderie at work to more intimate and focused interactions with a chosen few—in life. I now find myself tending a handful of friendships with great care, giving each a much higher priority in terms of time and planning than I ever gave friends and colleagues as a group. As I consider this transition, I am reminded of one of the byproducts of the brain changes neuroscientist Francine Benes studied: we seem to need less generic social activity—less affirmation from a group we are part of—than we did. That is surely so for me.

Taking Financial Care of Yourself

I am much further along in the personal fulfillment department than in the personal finance department. As my friends one by one come upon circumstances that require making informed decisions—even life-and-death decisions—about money, I worry about how fast I can catch up. Like many of us I have cherished the "room of one's own" part of Virginia Woolf's call for self-fulfillment without being aware that her formula was "*money* and a room of her own." In fact, Woolf devoted more of the book-length essay *Three Guineas* to the money part. She insisted that financial dependence and inexperience with money matters made it impossible for women to participate in the world as full citizens. The message, one we still need to hear, is that money, and the ability to handle it, is liberating on all levels. Without it, a room of one's own is only another prison.

Half a century later, another woman laid it on the line in no uncertain terms. "From fourteen to forty, [a woman] needs good looks, from forty to sixty she needs personality, and I'm here to tell you that after sixty she needs cash," advised Mary Kay Ash (taking off from a Sophie Tucker one-liner), who was forty-five when she started the cosmetics company that became the largest direct seller of skin-care products in the United States.

The biggest single obstacle to recalibrating our work life and making important decisions about how we spend our time is financial instability; the second biggest obstacle is lack of sophistication about money management. We are all painfully aware that the national and global economies intensify these realities: three quarters of employed women earn less than $30,000 a year, and the average pension for a woman is half that of a man, to mention just two sobering statistics. But despite widely varying degrees of expertise and confidence, we are trying to make important decisions about our financial future. There is no way around it. Before moving on, every one of us simply *must* become familiar with the underpinnings of our income—the nature of any investments we have, the requirements of our budgets, the appropriateness of our insurance and benefits, and the reliability or availability of advisors. In fact, unless a woman can project a middling income, the choices of Second Adulthood may be a luxury she cannot afford.

In an effort to get a grip on their finances, millions of women across the country have signed up for money management courses and guides. Typical is *Women Stuff,* a book that offers nuts-and-bolts advice about investment and surfing the web for financial information as well as discussions of prenups, divorce, and widowhood and, further on, a section entitled "Are we still awake?" Millions more women tune in for advice from Suze Orman, and other financial gurus, while still others have formed their own self-taught investors clubs. All these women are gaining expertise, but confidence often lags behind. Shelly, a talent agent and mother of a grown son, is no slouch in the money management department. For thirty years she has kept the books for her husband's business as well as her own. She has renegotiated their mortgages and reconfigured their stock portfolio. Nevertheless, when her husband's business took at dip at the same time she was trying to sell hers, she lost her cool. All her experience and her solid record of shrewd management gave way to a nightmare she thought she had outgrown. "I lay awake every night in a cold sweat," she told me. "I kept picturing us out on the street with nothing but a few shopping bags full of clothes. I thought I had outgrown the bag lady syndrome, but it was back."

The *bag lady syndrome* is a lurking fear among women Shelly's (and my) age, fear of waking up one day without the resources to take care of ourselves. No matter how much financial know-how we have, how much success we have, or how much or how little money we have, or where it comes from, we are vulnerable. Oprah Winfrey, one of the nation's top business-women, self-empowerment guru, and multimillionaire, told *Fortune* magazine that she once kept $50 million in cash as her "bag lady fund."

In Ruth and Karen's Retirement or What Next groups, every single woman admitted to a fear of waking up penniless. "Each one thinks it's her secret," Karen says. "And it paralyzes us. It can keep us in crappy jobs, crappy marriages, doing stuff we hate. It's a tyrant. We hear a voice saying, 'You're not going to make it if you leave this job, this marriage . . . whatever.'"

The bag lady syndrome is part long-term memory. It wasn't so long ago—before credit and divorce reform and job discrimination legislation changed the picture somewhat—that Gloria Steinem accurately pointed out that most married woman with kids were "one man away from welfare." It is part residue from our dream of a white knight who would carry us off to lifelong security—and the rude awakening that those knights often ride off into the sunset without us. Finally, it's part ambivalence about money itself. Many women were taught, on the one hand, that a woman was *too good* to concern herself with money—her devotion to her family was a calling beyond monetary measure—and, on the other hand, that we were *not good enough* brainwise to handle numbers. (This misconception was named "math anxiety" by author Sheila Tobias: the self-doubting assumption on the part of a student that even if she got a math problem right, it was by accident and would never happen again, because she simply didn't have a "math mind.")

Thank goodness, our daughters don't even recognize the term. When I asked my twenty-six-year-old researcher to check out the bag lady syndrome, she gave me a blank look; the notion of irrational money worries just didn't make sense to her.

Her generation is much more conversant with money matters and less emotionally confused. And the generation after hers is going to be even more confident. Many girls' schools and women's colleges now consider financial literacy a requirement and have designed courses that include everything from computing the interest on a credit card bill to filling out tax forms.

Sometimes we collaborate in our own ignorance. Sally, a devoted community volunteer, told me that throughout her twenty-year first marriage, her husband sat next to her when she signed their joint tax return with his hand over the section that totaled their income. "He said he didn't want me to worry about our investments," she explained. Her second husband is a little more forthcoming. She is beginning to understand— and, yes, worry about—their investments, but she feels less insecure than when the family finances were a mystery and she was "being taken care of." Beatrice, a successful administrator, has kept the household checkbook throughout her thirty-year marriage, but when her husband tries to explain the way their savings are being invested, her "eyes glaze over," she admits. It is she—not some sexist spouse—who "doesn't want to bother her pretty little head about money."

Even a career businesswoman can fall apart when it comes to putting a dollar value on her own work. One woman I met had been in the financial world her entire life and she knew she had top skills, but when she became a consultant, she was afraid to charge too much for her time. "Men do not have that problem," she observed. "They have a business card; they are a 'consultant.' It's $250 an hour, and that's that!" Another self-employed woman plays tricks on herself—and the bag lady. She has authorized her bank to send her a paycheck every month from her nest egg account. "Most of the time I don't need it, because I've got work," she says. "And then I'll just turn around and send it back. But since I'm so panicked all the time, I like the idea of 'okay, here's my salary.'"

"Money management is a skill," insists therapist Ruth Neubauer. "It's not that you can't do it; you just haven't. When you say 'I don't know how to do that,' you're saying 'there's something wrong with me.' It's a deficit model. But you can learn this like you have learned anything else in your life. It's not incapacitating. You don't have to stay terrified of this." Like the other terrifying leaps we find ourselves taking in Second Adulthood, this one can take us beyond fear. David Bach, who wrote the best selling advice book *Smart Women Finish Rich,* has observed how empowering the learning experience can be. "Once a woman learns how to take charge of her finances, she will never go back," he writes in a new introduction to his book. But that's only half the story. "The growing financial empowerment of women is not a fad," he adds, ". . . and it is going to change our destiny." Take that, bag lady!

Sheer Numbers: Our Secret Weapon Against the Inhospitable Workplace

The continuing empowerment of women in the workplace is a major factor in our changing destiny. In our generation, women who worked outside the home became the norm for the first time since industrialization replaced agriculture as the major workplace. Two-paycheck families became common, and it has been rare for a couple to get along on one throughout most of our adult life. Those continuously employed women, with their evolving expectations for their work future, are being joined in the job market by a growing population of newly-single widows and divorced women who are desperately in need of money and a sense of mission in their lives, and by those with later-in-life ambitions and new diplomas who are eager to use their new skills. Sara Rix, a senior policy analyst for AARP, attributes our unprecedented presence in the labor market to several economic factors—maintaining health care, recouping some retirement investments, getting social security benefits into the highest possible bracket—as well as one that is unique to our generation: "You have a lot of professional, skilled, middle-aged women," she points out, "who are saying that they are at the peak of their careers."

Despite our diverse goals, training, and motives, we are forming a critical mass in the workforce. As our numbers continue to rise, the participation of men in our age group is dropping. In fact, ours is the *only* group experiencing job growth during the recent recession. That numerical heft is our hidden strength. It establishes us as a force to be contended with by the very institutions that are currently making the workplace inhospitable to women of our age and with our employment history.

The typical work environment is inflexible and impatient, and ageist attitudes marginalize seasoned workers. Younger workers are ambitious and energetic, we are told, and learn faster. Furthermore, it is assumed that they "get" the technology. I can't tell you how many women described picking up an undercurrent of contempt every time they needed computer help or tried to produce a "visual" as flashy as a younger colleague's. Or, God forbid, they stopped into someone's office rather than e-mailing. As one woman, who has "sent out so many resumes my head is spinning," reports, "I am a physically fit, attractive, young-looking, energetic, and bright female with so much to offer a company, but somehow I feel this age discrimination thing is what's facing me for the first time in my life."

Even those who have good jobs are acutely aware that whatever financial security they have established is extremely precarious. Our salaries lag behind men's, and in a tight economy, benefits are cut back, a greater problem for women than for men, because we live longer. This is particularly threatening for the growing population of divorced women (over two million) who outnumber widows in the fifty to fifty-nine age group by two to one. (The numbers become more equal in the next decade.) Many of them lost access to their husbands' pensions in the divorce settlement, and many who had stayed home to raise children, find themselves behind in building for retirement in the jobs they took to support themselves. Recent economic downturns are forcing employers to retrench. The last-hired, first-fired layoffs are joining the replace-dead-wood-with-new-wood attitude toward older workers, destabilizing the already shaky employment picture for Second Adulthood women.

What We Have to Sell

But the very qualities we are beginning to discover about ourselves—the flexibility and "mellowness" to roll with the punches, growing confidence in our own judgment, and a newfound commitment to harmonizing our public and private values—will have a place in the workplace our generation is still redefining. Popular author of books about women's experience Naomi Wolf is cofounder of the Woodhull Institute (named after Victoria Woodhull, the nineteenth century feminist, stockbroker, and presidential candidate) which is dedicated to training the next generation of women leaders. To be successful in the world of the future, Wolf told me, young women will need to recognize and emulate certain qualities in their older colleagues: "The ability to think long-term not just short range; to factor emotional considerations, family toll, or opportunity into any given decision; to (compared to men of the boomer generation) leave ego outside the door when it is important to get things done on a practical level; to lead from a holistic perspective (taking into account the environment or human resources), not just see a reductive bottom line."

Ken Dychtwald, Ph.D., and author of *Age Power: How the 21st Century Will Be Ruled by the New Old,* is a gerontologist who sees those virtues working for us right now. "Boomer women," he told a teleconference of executives I attended, "have higher education and empowerment; they are the most amazing women our country has ever seen!" He urges personnel directors to focus on attracting, retraining, and creating benefits (particularly flexible hours) for us. Their companies can only benefit, he says, from the qualities older women are prepared to offer.

The very fact that many women approaching retirement age don't want to leave is a godsend, he asserts. It is more cost-effective to retain them; employee benefits take less from the bottom line than retirement benefits, which are accumulating at an alarming rate. (The Ford Motor Company is fast approaching the point where it will have more retirees than active workers.) Retraining is a better investment in an older employee than a younger, more ambitious one who will take the newly acquired skills and run, leaving the old-timers, if there are any left, to pass on the necessary know-how. Moreover, younger workers are in short supply compared to baby boomers, the largest demographic generation ever. Harder to pin down, but meaningful nonetheless, is our "zest" for work, combined with a more philosophical attitude toward moving up the ladder. Then there's all that experience—life and otherwise. One explanation of the unprecedented job growth for our group despite widespread unemployment is that employers can count on us to "be there and get the job done, perhaps better than someone who is younger and dealing with a lot more of life's hassles," says Jared Bernstein, of the Economic Policy Institute in Washington.

And then there are those famous *people skills.* The next wave of business growth, Dychtwald reminds his audiences, is going to be in the service sector, and while young people may be technological whizzes, "customer relations are not their strong suit," he points out wryly. Every day there are new findings about women's particular ability to pick up unspoken messages from others, form friendship networks, and promote harmonious interactions. Those attributes will become increasingly sought after as the economy becomes more dependent on cooperative work structures and informational and service products.

To the carrots of these advantages Dychtwald adds a stick that may come down on obtuse employers: "Older workers have gotten a bum rap. This is going to change. Boomers are going to start getting fired and they are going to sue and sue and sue and get so violent that employers are simply going to have to cut it out." Indeed, the number of age discrimination complaints brought before the Equal Employment Opportunity Commission rose over 24 percent between 2000 and 2002, making ageism the fastest growing category of discrimination cases.

It is clear that given our attitude and given our numbers, we are going to continue changing the workplace as our generation has been doing for the last thirty years. But the question for some of us is: do I want to keep bucking the system?

Going It Alone

Our record is impressive: We fought discrimination in the workplace and popularized the notion of family leave and flexible work schedules; we forced our way into institutions and professions and levels of leadership that even the most optimistic didn't dare predict happening in one generation. But for many, enough activism is enough. They want to stop fighting the system and invest their energies in themselves. For others, the shifting priorities of Second Adulthood are propelling them toward going it alone.

Women are starting new businesses at twice the national rate. They are the largest growing small (and some are *very* small) business sector in the economy and the source of the most newly created jobs. More surprising, an estimated two-thirds of the 6.2 million women business owners are over forty-five. (A little over half these business are—as might be expected—in the service sector, but the largest growing segment is in non-traditional industries, led by construction). To this endeavor we bring a lifetime of seat-of-the-pants problem solving, a recently acquired Fuck You Fifties sense of adventure, and a healthy dose of self-knowledge. On top of that we call upon our all-purpose survival tactic—networking.

Older entrepreneurs "are very resourceful," says a retired executive who has mentored several first-time businesses. "If they don't have the knowledge themselves, they find those that do. I think they are more sophisticated in that area than younger businesswomen. They are better able to recognize their own strengths and weaknesses and to find resources for the areas where they need support." Many entrepreneurs don't leave that crucial support to chance; they are forming small groups of women with a particular mix of expertise and a plan. "We help each other design marketing pieces for customers," says one member. "Business growth is the number one concern on the top of the minds of many entrepreneurs." These so-called *success teams* set goals and exchange know-how, ego-support, and referrals. They are doing for businesswomen what days on the golf course and in the locker room have done for men all these years. Actually, it's what women have been doing for each other in other areas all along. "There are days when you ask yourself what you are doing this for and if you are nuts," says Linda Hollander, author of *Bags to Riches: 7 Success Secrets for Women in Business.* "Your team is there to assure you that you are not."

Measured in numbers, the success rate of women business owners is impressive. According to *Business Week,* their collective sales now "surpass $1 trillion thanks to growth rates that continue to exceed national business averages . . . They employ a third again more people than the Fortune 500 and boast better loan repayment records. If anecdotal evidence in any indication, they also treat their employees better." For better or for worse, they also only pay themselves three-quarters of what men business owners do.

The real payoff for the woman entrepreneur is the chance to control her work life and, just as important, her work *style.* "A lot of women choose to be entrepreneurs in order to have control over their choices, not only so they can have other things in their lives, but also so the values and the business that they are in can be under their control," says consultant Carole Hyatt. Some of those values reflect gender differences between male- and female-run businesses that speak to the satisfactions of Second Adulthood. A study by the Center for Women's Business Research concluded that while "women and men entrepreneurs agree that there is more to success than monetary gain . . . Men entrepreneurs describe success in terms of gaining self-satisfaction for a job well done and achieving desired goals." Women, on the other hand, "derive satisfaction and success from building relationships with customers and employees, having control over their own destiny, and doing something they consider worthwhile."

In *Chapters,* a book about career change, Candice Carpenter, a cofounder of iVillage.com, describes a "moment of total clarity" in which she realized it was time to take control of her professional destiny and become an entrepreneur. She was at American Express, heading a group that was "doing a great job and having lots of fun" when an executive in the neighboring office told her that he had asked that her group be moved because their "laughter was distracting his team." She was stunned. "For me, humor was one of the most important survival skills in the work world . . . It would be two years before I finally left the company . . . But at that moment the pod that is me took off from the mother ship that was American Express and never came back."

Easing Out of the Workplace—by Degrees

As we reshuffle our priorities, and work moves down the list for many, a flexible or reduced schedule is the most desirable way to make room for the rest of life, and still stay connected to our skills and a steady paycheck. If consultants like Dychtwald have an impact, businesses will increasingly take advantage of the talent pool of Second Adulthood women. Right now 20 percent of employed women between forty-five and sixty-nine are working part time. For many that is a financial hardship, but for others it is the best offer around. Carol Atwood, a dynamic forty-nine-year-old entrepreneur, employs five thousand part-timers in her marketing business, and about half of them are her age or older. They recognize, she says, "that if you don't have flexibility to build other things into your life, time slips away and you haven't made your life meaningful. You haven't made it enriched, and you haven't had the spectrum of opportunity that you really require and hunger for." Of course, she adds, there is a trade-off: many of those older employees are "wildly overqualified."

Many formerly employed women who never want to "go to work" again a day in their lives insist that they don't want to stop "working" altogether. But when they contemplate volunteer work, they come up against a cultural bias already familiar to homemakers: voluntary work is seen as a lower form of productivity. Because women's unpaid work—both inside and outside the home—is not factored into the gross domestic product (though formulas have been developed that would make the calculation easy to do), the message is that it is of no value to the society as a whole. (The only time a homemaker's contribution takes on a dollar-and-cents value is if she dies and a court needs to figure out how to compensate her husband for the loss of her services.) The prospect of not being able to participate in *worthwhile* work is one of the reasons that many women I talked to are reluctant to retire—even if they could afford to.

A dynamic new organization in the New York area called The Transition Network (TTN) is composed of professional women who are, by choice or circumstance, easing into retirement. A survey of their membership showed that 70 percent saw "sustaining a sense of achievement" as a major concern, 55 percent chose "having fun," and 45 percent wanted to replace the sense of identity and structure that a workplace offers. For all of them, the biggest challenge is plugging into a source of collective professional energy. Their approach could be called the tend-and-befriend response—supportive and collaborative networking.

Redefining Volunteer Work

TTN offers support groups centering on particular concerns, circulates important information about work opportunities, health insurance, and financial planning, and is experimenting with "new models of work." A top priority of the organization is to reinvent volunteering. "Volunteer organizations don't know what to do with women like us," says Susan Ralston, a former book editor. "It's either 'do a benefit' or 'stuff envelopes'; or they feel so threatened that you can do what they do, but can do it for free, that they don't want to know from you." An alternative model that the group is testing is to "isolate a project and go in as if you were a consulting team, only you are working pro bono. You go in, you do the project, and you get out and go on to the next project." That way the work is a good match with the volunteers' skills, and the salaried staff isn't threatened.

Retirement (or "*rewire*ment" as it is called by the authors of *Don't Retire, Rewire*—an approach to self-discovery and reinvention) is being redefined by groups like The Transition Network, as well as by every woman who sees her decision to retire in a different way. A sixty-three-year-old women's studies professor described her outlook this way in *Women Confronting Retirement: A Nontraditional Guide,* a collection of experiences edited by Nan Bauer-Maglin and Alice Radosh: "Retirement . . . was a chance to shift from work to the self, from responsibility to freedom . . . I could turn my attention to the neglected areas of my life where repair and reclamation were still possible."

A shift from work to the self is how the recalibration of the time/money/satisfaction equation feels. Whether a woman is retiring, like the professor who is concentrating on "repair and reclamation," or whether she is preparing to "go off like a rocketship," like the executive emerging from a professional holding pattern, she is not the worker she was, only older. In many ways, she is not a worker any more at all. The ingredients may be the same ones that have motivated us in the past, but we don't necessarily crave them in the same proportion. Indeed, work as we have known it will not be the be-all-and-end-all for us; our real work lies in our lives as a whole, which may or may not include "work." And tending our fields of dreams.

CHAPTER SIX

Rediscovering Your Passion, Facing Your Fear

"There is a vitality, a life force, an energy, a quickening that is translated through you into action, and because there is only one of you in all time, this expression is unique. And if you block it, it will never exist through any other medium and it will be lost. The world will not have it. It is not your business to determine how good it is or how valuable nor how it compares with other expressions. It is your business to keep it yours clearly and directly, to keep the channel open."

—Martha Graham, quoted by Agnes DeMille, *Martha: The Life and Work of Martha Graham*

As the commitment to work loses intensity and as family ties loosen with circumstance, we are in a position to close in on our deepest drives, our passions. What *really* matters. Which is not to say that clarity comes with opportunity. When I attended a Transition Network meeting where fifty women were asked who had a passion they wanted to pursue, only two hands went up. The rest of us looked on enviously. We had lists of possibilities in our minds, but we were awaiting the promptings of the heart. All of us long to make contact with that unique inner drive that fuels our most important decisions. Much of what happens in the Fertile Void feels like an archeological dig in search of it. Passion is the "postmenopausal zest" we hope will inspire the choices we make about work, money, relationships, and how we spend the rest of our lives.

Yet it is hard to recognize, more so in oneself than in another. It is clear to me that Rita's passion is languages; "I'm so excited by languages," she told me more than once. I am sure that whatever else she does with her Second Adulthood, she will make a place for her love of languages and take satisfaction and energy from that commitment. Yet when she took a find-your-dream workshop, she couldn't identify an abiding passion. Only at the end of our conversation did Rita become aware that her life story had a very clear and persistent pulse to it that was already beginning to nourish her Second Adulthood. Like many of us, she dismissed the steady pilot light burning in her soul; she thinks of passion as something that sweeps you off your feet.

No Two Are Alike

I have friends whose passions are clear. One, a writer, can become so transported by her work that sometimes when I call, she hardly recognizes my voice. Another has played tennis almost every morning at 7 A.M. for thirty years, wearing out numerous partners along the way—she loves the sport that much. For many people I know, music is the ingredient that makes life worth living, enhancing the good moments, and assuaging the bad. For Margo, the executive-turned-Peace-Corps-volunteer, the only downside to her two years in Africa was limiting her weekly ballet classes to every six months when she came home on a visit. My politically committed friends think nothing of staying up all night hammering out a position paper; indeed, they draw energy from the intensity of the experience. I envy them. I envy their ability to lose a sense of time and place when they are engaged in pursuing What Matters to them.

I can recognize passion when I see it, but I have a hard time feeling it. I love to paint and occasionally lose track of time when I am at it, yet I don't get to it very often. I love to ski and feel transported with exhilaration when I am on the slopes, but getting there always seems too complicated. What I have always loved is my work, but I was too busy working to explore what part of that work really got my juices going. Now, with the clarity of the Fertile Void, I see what aspect I couldn't live without: If I never earned another penny at it, what matters to me is trying to figure out what is going on with the people around me and putting what I have discovered into words. Indeed, I would do this anyway, in my mind, as I do traveling on a train or sitting in a café, even if I never had the opportunity to set the words to paper. The passion is the watching and thinking; the joy is expressing the results. However, along with the joy comes fear, fear that I will make a fool of my presumptuous self by going public with my work. Still, that is what I would go out of my way to do—even get up early for. For me, that's passion.

It's no roaring conflagration. It doesn't rule my life. I don't think I would give up everything else to pursue it. Until this moment, I wouldn't have described myself as someone with a passion to figure out people in words. Yet, from now on, I will think of this as my pilot light. Too often we think Second Adulthood passion has to involve finding a new job or learning a whole new skill or traveling to new places. All those things can be fun and enrich our lives, but the real thing is not necessarily that easy to tap—or even that radical.

We've all got dreams and drives; the hard part is accessing them. For some, like Rita with her love of languages, the passion is familiar but overlooked. For others, like me, it is obscured by the daily grind and a belief that only other people have it. For still others, it is out there—unconnected to any experience so far—and needs to be reeled in. "Is there any totally off-the-wall idea that comes into your mind when you think of what you'd like to do next?" I asked Betty, who found her no! during her son's year-long illness. We were at the end of a long conversation about her readiness to take off—but to where? A contributing factor to her sense of possibility was (here Virginia Woolf would smile knowingly) a small inheritance she had received when her ninety-seven-year-old father died. "I had my own money for the first time. It gave me a sense of security . . . and a sense of power that I'd never had before."

Still, she wasn't able to particularize that sense of power. She had run through an array of interests that had bubbled up after she retired from teaching. She had written a novel for preteens and put it away years earlier when it was rejected by just one publisher. She had loved those months of writing every day and she was determined to get back to it. "If I set certain times, I could say to people who ask me to do things, 'I'm sorry that's my writing morning,' which I haven't been willing to do so far because I don't think I really felt that I had the right to say that." She told me how she had taken several drawing classes in the past and still really wanted to learn to draw. "Jane Austen is one of my favorite novelists," she explained. "Every woman in those days could sketch. She could make a 'likeness.' The heroines were 'gifted,' but everyone could do it . . . If I could get to the point where I could sketch a little bit, I think that would give me a lot of pleasure." And she told me about how she was sure she could "design the best suitcase." She and her son have half-humorously discussed starting a business. "I am an expert on suitcases," she admits. "I was one of the first non-airline people to get the ones with little wheels . . ."

As we reviewed these projects, it was clear that she was motivated by them, but her energy only peaked when I invited her to think off-the-wall. "I really would like to do something with animals," she said in a rush of words. "I could see myself getting involved with animal rescue work. That really appeals to me." Something in her voice suggested that she was scaring herself. I only began to understand why this was such a daring dream when she talked about how she saw herself in it. "A little bit in the wild, with animals," adding "I don't usually see myself as a wild person." She then recalled marching in anti-war demonstrations in the sixties. "I like that image of myself. Besides that, I've really not been much of a crusader. Maybe I could write a book indoctrinating children against animal cruelty . . . I don't see myself doing anything violent, but maybe I could do it with my pen." She had found what she had been searching for all along—not the project, but the passion. And it was accompanied by fear.

Do I Really Want to Get Carried Away?

The prospect of becoming possessed by an irrational force is frightening. The word passion itself is frightening. Most women associate it with the unknown territory of being out of control, following our irrational instincts, or being totally and neglectfully self-involved. We also associate it with another taboo—anger, real killer anger. And most women are reluctant to go there. Or have been. As the journey unfolds, many women are finding that confronting a lifetime of resentments, disappointments, and feuds—with Fuck You Fifties defiance—can release all kinds of energy, including, for some, the passion that was thwarted by contempt or by neglect from someone important.

The word is also heavily laden with sexual connotations. It's not as though we got through our first half century—let alone the 1950s (and 1960s, for that matter)—without some serious hang-ups about wild abandon. So maybe we need a less laden word. "Juices," as in "getting your juices going," is a wholesome-sounding term that came up in my conversations. Several women spoke about finding their whimsy—impulsive flights of fancy—after a lifetime of everything but.

Those words evoke a carefree spontaneity that some are beginning to experience when playing with their grandchildren, but the rest of us can hardly remember. We are mired in our more structured and literal-minded first adulthood. Playfulness is a bridge back to the time when we were most free. Carol Gilligan and others have pointed out that to get a glimpse of who we can become in our Second Adulthood, we need to find our way back to the spirited ten- and eleven-year-olds we once were when our passions were more accessible.

The prospect of reaching your inner child by accessing playful abandon can be as much fun as trying to learn to belly dance while wearing a girdle. Ridiculous. Feeling foolish and looking ridiculous as we experiment with new emotional outlets are experiences we are sure we don't need right now. It is hard enough to keep our dignity in the face of so many disconcerting developments. But Dr. George E. Vaillant, a Harvard gerontologist, insists that as we age, we can and should expose ourselves to silliness. In his scheme of things, play is not a frivolous pursuit at all, but an important "guidepost to a happier life." The trick, he offers, is "learning how to maintain self-respect while letting go of self-importance." In his book *Aging Well*, he celebrates the exhilaration of play after a lifetime of goal-oriented activity; it "produces joy, and joy requires neither reinforcement or reward." We have experienced our share of rewards. Joy—which is passion played out—is one of the adventures available in Second Adulthood.

Play also produces laughter. Laughter has the characteristics—getting carried away, blurting out inanities, losing control—of other emotional surges, but without the "dangers." When was the last time you laughed so hard you couldn't breathe? Therapist Ilana Rubenfeld, who coined the phrase "fertile void," calls humor a "martial art," because it combats fear. Laughter, like sex, affects the body by "stimulation followed by relaxation." In addition, laughter "improves blood circulation, increases the oxygenation of the blood, enhances digestion, reduces pain (because of the release of endorphin, the brain's own pleasure-producing energy), and best of all strengthens the immune system." Rubenfeld recommends starting, if you must, with a fake smile. "The very act of lifting the corners of the mouth—'mouth yoga'—affects our body chemistry and makes us feel better," she explains. This really works. I do a few exaggerated fake smiles as I ride the stationary bicycle every morning, and I am here to tell you it lifts the spirits. It also disconcerts those working out around me, which satisfies my Fuck You Fifties sense of mischief and makes me smile for real. Better yet, get your inner circle of friends together and tell each other what made you laugh yourself silly, whenever it was. Then, after you've been on-the-floor laughing, let loose some of your off-the-wall dreams.

The two stories that follow are as unique as the passions in each woman. One is about passion lost in work and the other is about passion found in work. Joanne found her energies radically refocused onto her awakening physicality after a lifetime of living in her head. Joanie found her power for the first time by taking an unpremeditated and frightening "plunge." For each of them an inner power surge was detonated by saying yes when no was the appropriate response. Both use the word *joy* to describe what was added to their lives. It is there in each of us, too.

JOANNE'S STORY
"I Could Swoosh Down and Then Come Back Up
and Not Get Dizzy. It Is Just a Magical Thing"

Although she grew up in the South, Joanne is the antithesis of stereotypical Southern womanhood: she is open, earnest, and very no-frills. Her bearing, as she settles herself in an armchair in her blindingly sunny one-bedroom apartment, suggests a stoic pioneer woman. Until recently, her life had been driven by a powerful force; she called it a passion, but ultimately it stopped nourishing her.

"I'm not sure where my save-the-world passion came from," she begins. "Maybe it was wanting to save myself as an unhappy kid, and then wanting to save the world because if other people were unhappy, I understood that and wanted to save them, too. . . ." She remembers her school-age self as "very much a person who lived in her head and sort of escaped through books. When I was in college I was more interested in politics than I was in the dances. That had something to do with that I was in college in Mississippi in the 1960s, and the politics were infinitely more interesting."

She has always lived alone. Politics and social activism and her work for a human rights lobby were her whole life. "It was hard work, but it was fun, all the marches and the political strategizing." Her friends were from work, social life outside of work was nil, and her sense of accomplishment came from the collective process. It was like that until she turned forty. One day, a colleague dared Joanne—considered notoriously unathletic among her friends—to join her in signing up for a fitness class. Always ready to serve, she took the six-week program and, lo and behold, "I could touch my toes! And I learned that I could do those things, and I could improve."

At the same time—as a result?—she began to feel "burned out. That I wasn't doing enough for myself. I don't think I could have articulated it then, but I was trying hard to realize that if you give yourself away all the time, there's nothing left. It's in my nature to give myself all away." Like many of us, when she began to recalibrate her work life, she found that her priorities had shifted. Serving others was about to be pushed off the top of the list.

To begin paying attention to herself, she requested a three-month sabbatical, and Joanne began researching not the Grand Tour, but adventure programs. She was saying no to everything that had been expected of a self-sacrificing and well-brought-up Southern lady. She scoured the outdoor magazines (this was before the Internet) and settled on an environmental group that organized projects in exotic places. It was quite a leap. She had never traveled alone—"never even really taken vacations"—and had only recently begun to test her physical prowess. "I didn't have a clue if I could do it," she admits. Nevertheless, driven by some inner force she couldn't identify, she took herself off on three rugged trips—hiking in New Zealand and Australia and an Earthwatch project in Bali. "We went to all the shadow puppet plays and we were up all night . . . and I learned to use one of those reel-to-reel tape recorders," she exults. "And I met some really nice people."

Until then, Joanne realizes now, she "didn't have anything else going on in my life *except* my work. All day, every day, including weekends. It was like a gift to me to realize that there were other things. And when I came back, I kept up the physical activity. It made me more alert and more energetic and better able to do my work, which was still my purpose in life."

Soon after she turned fifty, several things happened. The organization she worked for went under, and the workplace family members that had been so intimately supportive were forced to go their separate ways. It was wrenching, but Joanne managed to find a job in which she dealt with social policy—more save-the-world work. But, she realized, "I didn't have a new family, just a new job."

Up to this point, her shifting commitment that was revealing itself as an awakening of her body had given Joanne an energizing new hobby, but it took a stroke of fate to kindle her real passion. One day when she went to the Y to work out, there was a long wait for the bikes, and she decided to check out what else was going on. She stumbled into a class called NIA (Neuromuscular Integrative Action). "There were a lot of people in there, and they were barefoot, and there was great music, and people were laughing! I'd never seen anybody laugh in an aerobics class." She went in "all dressed up in my shoes and socks" and tried it. "People would go across the room and then they'd come back and then they would free dance. I felt like I had three left feet, and I was going to leave, but"—ever the well-mannered lady—"I didn't want to just walk out in the middle. I didn't think that would be very polite. So I stayed. And by the end of class I still couldn't do it, but it captured me somehow." She had literally stumbled into Dr. Vaillant's life-enhancing insight about play. "There was a joy in that room," she says simply.

It was three months before she took her shoes off, because she couldn't believe she was making a commitment to dance, of all things. "I remember the moment when I first realized I could swoosh down and then come back up and not get dizzy.

It is just a magical thing." Actually NIA is more than running around barefoot. It is a combination of three martial arts, yoga, various forms of body work, and jazz, modern, and Isadora Duncan dance movement. For Joanne this was a recipe for self-fulfillment. As she became "physically free," she flashed back to herself at five or six when she shut down her twirling and joyous self. "I remember what it was like to dance around the room and to twirl until you fell down and how great that felt." She was beginning to connect the pieces of her life, the child and the adult, the intellectual and the physical.

She also connected to some deep emotions. "Some of the moves brought up some things that I didn't quite understand and in fact still don't understand, although I went into therapy and explored them, that were really scary. Anger. And sadness. I had never given myself permission to be sad. But with the way your body moves with music, it's hard to censor feelings like that."

Joanne's commitment to NIA brought her into a new family, one that for the first time in her life, had no connection to work. Many of her friends are much younger than she is and have exposed her to new ways of looking at the world. The evening I interviewed her, she was going to the home of a woman whose mother had died recently and who wanted all her friends around when she described their last days together. "It was not tragic," Joanne says her friend told her; "there was joy, too." Those friends—along with a core of friends from her earlier life—sustained Joanne through the souring of her job experience and her efforts to set up her own consulting business.

By now the work/life balance of her existence has shifted. Her NIA training is the linchpin, the passion, the focus of her energies. She is working toward the teaching level and enjoys her newfound community. Her consulting business provides income and clients—but not close friends—and makes it possible to regularly take a day or two off for NIA training. She has to be disciplined about time. Because she is so passionate about devoting herself to dancing, she has gotten a lot better about saying no when in the past it would have been easier—or more polite or more "giving"—to say yes.

Joanne's days give her a sense of harmony—and authenticity—that she has never experienced before. She is more passionate and, at the same time, more mellow. Her save-the-world drive has abated a bit, and is still the major satisfaction of her work—but her work is not her whole life. "Now I also care about what I can learn or how I can improve my flexibility or posture, even though I am as old as I am. And I also care about spending time with friends who don't spend a lot of time talking about saving the world. I'm just more laid-back than I ever was." She has added one more precious dimension to her life. "I spend more time with my nieces, which I really love. They're at the stage in their lives where I was when I still loved twirling—before I lost it."

JOANIE'S STORY
"That's What I Like About Me—My Whimsy"

Joanie grew up in San Francisco in a wealthy family. She was an agreeable and accomplished young woman of twenty-six when she got married in 1978. From the start the marriage was a traditional one, with demanding in-laws, but she came up with some untraditional approaches to doing what was expected of her. For one thing, she kept her own name. "That's who I was," she says matter-of-factly. "It seemed ridiculous to me, when you get married, to change who you are." She got no objection from her husband, "maybe because he had been

married before . . ." When she took on the expected responsibilities of volunteer work, it was with a collective devoted
to medical rights for women. "They were all sort of hippies
then, but I always fit in somehow." And when she began to
join organization boards, she chose the American Civil Liber-
ties Union. As her family grew—she now has three children,
aged twenty-one, nineteen, and fourteen—she focused her
volunteer efforts on schools.

Her wife-and-mother adulthood now looks to her "sort of
like labor. Did I love labor? No. But the magic that comes out
of it makes you forget about the labor." Like Joanne, she is
aware of having become more laid-back with age. "When I
think back at what would unravel me then, it seems so silly. My
mother-in-law is now telling me how I wouldn't let my kids
have sugar for the first two years of their life. I said, 'Oh gosh,
I was so controlling.'"

She has begun to appreciate the process of letting go of regrets and of responsibilities. "I also realize that there was no
question of whether or not to have kids. I was part of the culture that said, 'You are not fulfilled without children.' So, was
I happy? I'm happy I did it. By the third one, I'm a better
mother. I love the human beings that they are. That's the glory
of now. It also helps me let go. I've given what I could. Now
let me watch them . . . and learn from them. That's where the
aging process helps—with letting go of control and being
freer."

On a totally out-of-character whim, she bought herself a
pied-à-terre in New York City, a four-hour train ride from
home. "It is my Second Adulthood home," she explains, everything a "room of one's own" should be. In fact, it was Joanie
who reminded me of the "enough money" part of the Woolf
quote; of all the women I interviewed, the one with the most

money had the most respect for the impact of having too little. Perhaps that is because she had spent much of her adult life giving it away, and observing the changes it could make.

The apartment of her own became "an escape . . . a kind of sanctuary. I came here for a break from my kids' teenagehood, from all the domesticity, and I loved it. I just felt like a free person." She decorated it in her own taste, a sort of Alice in Wonderland collection of odd-shaped furniture and her own photography. Her prize possession is a mirror stand that she commissioned from a craftswoman artist. It is carved and painted wood, decorated with phrases that have particular meaning for her, and they resonate with the Second Adulthood journey. Beneath the mirror are three commandments: "No need to sparkle," "No need to hurry," and "No need to be anybody but oneself."

She bought the apartment before she had any relationship to the modern dance company that has taken over her life. Yet having the apartment made it possible—even mystically necessary—to accept the assignment. Originally she and her husband had been solicited to join the board. He declined and she thought she would, too; the last thing she needed was another volunteer commitment. But while she thought she had made the decision to say no, a voice within was saying yes! "My daughter's a dancer," Joanie explains. "Since she was a little girl, we've had what we called 'private dates' going to dance concerts. I'd seen this company dance, and I remember being wowed." So she took her version of my Outward Bound step back off a cliff, and said, Yes!

"Honestly." She sighs. "I didn't know what I was getting into." The more she learned about the company, the more problems she saw for the board; but she was carried forward by "almost the whimsy of saying, 'yeah, why not?' And that was the beginning. I keep thinking of Gloria Steinem's book *Outrageous Acts and Everyday Rebellions,*" she explains. "She says, 'just do it.' Even if others think it's outrageous, if it feels like you, do it. I think what happens for me is that my mind kind of turns off, and the heart moves forward, and I plunge . . ."

In the three years since then, she has plunged over and over again. She agreed to become chair of the board and has become "an obnoxious fund-raiser." She has also learned to do something that terrified her—speak in public. When she despaired of being able to do that, she told herself, " 'What's the job? I'm going to do the job because I believe in what I'm doing.' It kind of frees you up if you believe in what you are doing. I asked myself, 'Do I need to succeed?' Well, I'm not going to fail. Because I can't fail this company."

Like many of us, she discovered that the more outspoken she became, the less distracted she was by her unspoken ideas—and the more ready to hear others. "As I'm getting more used to liking to hear my voice out there, I really want to hear other voices we haven't heard. Particularly people who don't want to speak—'I have nothing to say' or 'I'm only good in small groups'; it's amazing."

She also discovered that her commitment and her willingness to speak out has emboldened her to develop a leadership style. "I like a model that feels more akin to women, more collaborative. It's not against men, but it's against hierarchy. I think that parenting prepared me for this. How do I listen? Am I pushing too hard? Or not hard enough?" When she thinks about her power, she pauses. "Wherever I put my passion, that's my power."

Serious as the work is that she does from wherever she is, she experiences the joy of play on the several days a month she spends in her apartment. She makes her own schedule and is more outspoken and freewheeling. "I am more free and wild here," she says. But like so many of the recalibrations in Second Adulthood, Joanie's newfound commitment throws off some of the other components of her life. "The work is easy," she says. "Dealing with the relational changes is . . . horrible. All this," she says embracing her surroundings, "is changing the dynamic that we have as a couple, as a family. I also have a mother-in-law next door, so I get, 'You're going off to the city *again?*'"

She is finding the reinvention of her marriage especially stressful. "Realizing that your children really are able to stand on their own is one thing, but there is the obligation to your partner/spouse. I realize it's hard, because he envisioned, like most men, 'I'm getting ready to retire soon and now you're free and let's go. Aren't you going to follow me around the world?' but it's 'Let's go to my places.'" It will be hard to sort all this out, she says, but she is learning more about intimacy every day. "I don't blame my husband anymore for what he isn't or what it is I need, that perhaps I need to give to myself. And I now see and truly believe this man loves me for my passion."

Most of all, she is beginning to get to know her true self through the exercise of her passion. It is not being the chair of the board of a dance company, though that is a transforming life experience. What makes her special, what she has to offer to the people and projects she cares about is the quality she calls whimsy. By which she means, I finally figured out, the drive to follow her own gut feelings—her whims—and let her instincts find her passions. "That," she says, "is what I like about me. My whimsy."

———

When ignited, whether it is a pilot light or a blinding light, a passion illuminates the inner recesses of who we are. And whether its outlet is a hobby or a major commitment, passion is about letting go. No wonder it engenders fear. But like the lesson of my descent down the cliff wall, the response to fear can be yes! "Make your fears your agenda," a Jungian philosopher is reported to have told a patient. By that I think he meant that the experiences that had been relegated as off limits by fear were just the ones that held the most promise for discovery. And as Joanie and Joanne and so many women I talked to found, passion stands up to fear. Even the tiniest little passion is an authentic expression of curiosity about something out there in the world—that comes from in here, in each of us.

CHAPTER SEVEN

Redefining Intimacy

Love, Sex, Friendship, and the New You

*. . . This body
that's been sucked out like an egg.
But the heart has no notion
of time. It's not a cat
who poses aloof upon your return,
but a dog that leaps up
to slobber your face. No matter
that it's rummaged in garbage or
licked its own ass, it can't
conceive you wouldn't want it.*

—Ellen Bass, "Falling in Love At 55"

My adolescent daydreams about love stayed with me well into my first adulthood. The fact that they didn't come true only made them more romantic. My ideal was the doomed consuming passion of Heathcliff and Cathy in *Wuthering Heights*. When she cried out, in a paroxysm of anguish, "I *am* Heathcliff!" and he cried out later, in even greater anguish, "I cannot live without my life! I cannot live without my soul!"—my heart cried out, "Right on!"

I realized how far from that total-immersion view of intimacy I had come when a friend announced matter-of-factly, "I am going out of the emotional management business," and every cell of my being cried out *right on*. It is the idea of *not* being consumed by devotion that appeals to me now.

As we move through the Fertile Void, most of us long for the time and space to absorb and evaluate and experiment with what we are discovering. And as we become more grounded and confident, the pleasure of being a free agent is real. What matters now is the need for solitude and the joy of following one's own directives, and that runs counter to intimacy as we may have known it. But together these imperatives set the stage for what can work: a scaled-down devotion—an eagerness to share but not consume. These drives bring us to the frontier of a new kind of intimacy—tender and noninvasive—based on new priorities.

At the same time, bonds forged under the old terms may be demanding attention. Husbands who are retiring just as their wives are getting a second professional wind make emotional and caretaking demands—or offers of dream trips to exotic places—that can awaken the familiar push-pull of needs and priorities. So can children who are flocking back to the empty nest in times of economic or emotional need. So can ailing parents—in a big way.

In this particularly sensitive recalibration, the new priorities emerge from the discoveries of the journey so far. The first is *authority,* the power to find and assert one's true self. This is the force that sets off the Fuck You Fifties and picks up steam as we learn to count on it. The second priority is *space*—as in Virginia Woolf's *A Room of One's Own*—the recognition that each of us needs the nourishment of her own company. Like authority, breathing room is an acquired taste that becomes a life-giving force in Second Adulthood. When Rosalynn Carter was asked the secret of her long and productive marriage to the former president, she responded with an intensity that defied

her honey southern drawl: "Space!" You can get companionship and affection from others, we are learning, but not com-
pleteness.

The recalibration of intimacy may be one of the most confusing aspects of Second Adulthood, because each relationship
is unique, and the shift can be seismic or it can be impercepti-
ble. Friends may require special attention or may become
strangers. Partners can develop needs that must be met—illness,
for one—or challenged. Homemakers whose husbands have recently retired have been heard to say, "I married him for better
or for worse, but not for lunch!" At the same time, we are being forced by circumstances to reevaluate our responsibilities—
and the space we need—in relation to our children and to our
parents. As Joanie (the whimsical one) confessed with anguish,
even though the rest of her life was coming together in a joyous way, "dealing with the relational changes is horrible!"

One Plus One

The romantic equation has been tricky all along. If they ever
shared my Healthcliff–Cathy model, most women have outgrown it. We know that one plus one will never equal one.
Most of us have also learned that if one plus one turns out to
equal no more than two—a pair of people with no common
ground—intimacy is lacking. If all goes well during our first
adulthood, however, our most intimate relationships have taken
on a life of their own in which one plus one equals three—two
people, plus a unique creation between them with a dynamic
of its own. A couples' therapist I once knew explained that she
was treating not the partners but the overlap between them,
"the relationship." In Second Adulthood the focus shifts again,
to reconfiguring the parameters of that shared space. Having

spent most of our adult lives trying to overthrow *de*pendence and build up our resources of *in*dependence, we are ready to make what the late, great Bella Abzug once called "a declaration of *inter*dependence."

For me, the most successful area of new interdependence in my marriage is our social life; my husband and I now regularly make our own evening plans. We check with each other, of course, and we do lots of things together, but five or six years ago it would never have occurred to me to accept an offer to dinner or to a movie that was just for me. Circumstances made it easier to do this—no more childcare or evening homework to worry about—but the simple theory that we weren't joined at the hip took a while to take hold in practice. I am regularly reminded of how deeply entrenched the Noah's Ark mindset is when I invite a couple to dinner, and the wife says that they can't come because her husband has a meeting that night; she is taken aback by my suggestion that she come anyway. In her hesitation I recognize both the fear that she can't hold her own amid other couples and her worry that her husband will feel threatened by her socializing without him. Such emotions can make even the smallest adjustment in a long-term relationship traumatic.

Changing the rules can be a particularly alarming development for those in our lives who have counted on our devotion. Our revised priorities may feel like rejection. It is hard to reassure them that the new intimacy we are forging is based on creating a life-enhancing breathing space between us. Men in particular are more than a little bewildered by how we are redefining ourselves in relation to them. Since we know almost nothing about how this stage of life is affecting them, it is hard to anticipate how much they will panic at the prospect of the vacuum our "space" is creating in their lives. And how the changes boiling up inside us will affect the relationship that had endured under different terms.

The Hormone Factor

At every stage of our journey, the themes of Second Adulthood intersect in new ways, and the raging hormones that are a recurring motif can play an especially disruptive part in domestic upheaval. Christiane Northrup, author of the best-selling book *The Wisdom of Menopause,* discovered firsthand how loss of estrogen can play a role in stripping down an intimate partnership. In preparation for fibroid surgery she was given drugs that put her into temporary menopause quite quickly and a few years ahead of schedule. Soon after she began taking the medication, a perfectly innocent evening in front of the TV turned into a marital turning point. As they were watching *E.R.* her husband made a pronouncement about the medical profession—something he had done frequently before. Only this time, Dr. Northrup explained, she blew up. "After years and years of down-regulating my personal truth to make myself acceptable to my husband and to every authority figure like him in medical school," she writes, "I simply couldn't keep still another moment." The argument escalated, but instead of being more intimidated by his intransigence, she felt herself "grow taller and taller with my own truth." Everything spilled out—"what I believed, about medical practice, about our relationship, about the inequity in the way we'd been living all those years—and I offered no excuses for what I said, nor any attempt to make it easier to hear. . . . At the end my husband did not look as tall as he had at the beginning, and he was speaking softly and apologizing to me. That was the turning point in our marriage. There was no going back." She had established her own authority.

Even though this menopause was temporary, it precipitated her sojourn in the Fertile Void during which she began to explore her own space. "I put all my significant relationships under a microscope," she writes, "began to heal the unfinished business from my past, experienced the first pangs of the empty nest, and established an entirely new and exciting relationship with my creativity and vocation."

Change and Commitment

Joan and Robert Parker experienced the reallocation of space literally. Their story is one of trial and error. When their last child left home, they found their temperaments and lifestyle interests no longer compatible—she liked to socialize and stay up late; he liked to read at home and pack it in early—so they moved into separate apartments. But they still enjoyed one another's company and had no real animosity toward each other. After a couple of years, they tried another living arrangement— a large Victorian house with an apartment on the ground floor and an exterior stairway to another apartment on the top floor. He took the one with the larger kitchen because he's the cook. She took the garret because she's the romantic. Joan hardly ever uses the outside stairway, but it confirms her sense of freedom. They entertain together and separately and make their own schedules. They even began working together on TV scripts based on the detective novels he writes. Robert calls theirs "a loving, monogamous relationship." Joan calls it their "second marriage."

To Carolyn Heilbrun, in her classic book *Writing a Woman's*

Life, a benign midlife readjustment such as this becomes a re-marriage. In a good one, she wrote, "everything is debatable and challenged; nothing is turned into law and policy. The rules, if any, are known only to the two players, who seek no public trophies."

Circumstances can help ease the way. As the stresses of family and work recede, both personalities may drift toward a potentially companionable middle ground. The three macho drives—money, power, and sex—abate on his side, while directness, authority, and assertiveness rise on hers. But in a relationship that has become set in its ways, the redistribution of power is not easy.

The power imbalance I had felt in my marriage but never really defined for myself came into blinding focus when I came upon this description of a domestic dynamic in Mary Catherine Bateson's *Composing a Life:* "For at least twenty years, whenever I interrupted my husband when he was busy, he finished what he was doing before he responded. When he interrupted me, I would drop what I was doing to respond to him, automatically giving his concerns priority." Her words evoked the state of anxiety and suspended animation that I associated with being at home. How many times had I left a thought behind never to retrieve it, or left a task unfinished until I was too tired to do it right, or abandoned a plan to do something for myself—something as modest as getting my hair washed—because something for someone else had come up? Along with the anger that had periodically bubbled up over this inequity for over thirty years, I became aware of a more engaging insight: I had relinquished my power—and I could get it back. Not without a struggle, of course, from those who have become used to my snapping to attention. But every time I hear myself say, "I'll be with you when I'm done" or "I'm busy now, can we talk about that later," I feel my authority asserting itself. And every time I literally will myself to take the few minutes to do what I need or want to do, I breathe the freshness of a growing space between me and those I love.

Alexis, whose unintentional creation of the PISS acronym for her reinvention efforts prompted such a good laugh, says that she and her husband are "trying to refocus what we like to do together," but the "together" is harder to redefine than the "things we do." "We golf together and we hope to travel together, but we're still two very different people. I have this vision sometimes of us having to swim this huge lake to get together. . . . I'm thinking, 'I don't think I have the energy to make it to you, honey, on this one . . .'" But, she goes on, "occasionally we do meet, and it's great. We were high school sweethearts, so we've been through all stages of our lives together, and as boring as that may sound to many, it's great for us."

"Companionship," the simple pleasure in each other's company, is the term that comes up most often in connection with interdependence achieved after a long haul. Jenny had lived with Jay happily for twenty years, during which time they raised the five children they brought from previous marriages. When the children moved out and both cut back on their work, they were amazed to discover how much fun it was to "be together—doing errands, whatever!" So they decided to get married—not to cement their commitment to themselves or their children, but to commemorate the new companionate dimension in their relationship. Ironically, it was Hillary Clinton who best defined compatible intimacy for all of us who have been through the wars of a long-standing marriage: "All I know is that no one understands me better and no one can make me laugh the way Bill does," she wrote in answer to those who thought she was crazy not to leave him. "Bill Clinton and I started a conversation in the spring of 1971, and more than thirty years later we're still talking."

Hillary Clinton got past more than most women have to, but in my conversations with married women, I kept hearing the theme of "I just let it go more now." "I try not to waste time obsessing on the nuances of our marriage," said Beatrice. For her, letting go of shoulda-woulda-coulda brooding makes for reinvigorated authority. "At the same time I don't let him get away with stuff that ate me up inside because I was afraid to start a fight. We probably fight more now, but the fights are shorter and less devastating than they were. I just try to enjoy the good stuff. And the good stuff *is* good," she adds with a mischievous smile. She is among the many (46 percent, in one study) long-married women who find their sex life is better than ever. "Even though we don't have sex as often, when we do, we know we can count on each other to find ways to make it work. Sometimes it's really great; sometimes there are even surprises." She does have one big complaint. "The snoring. A cure for snoring would be bigger than Viagra—and would save more marriages, too!"

Moving On

Some marriages can't—and shouldn't—be saved. Many women need to literally walk away from their earlier lives in order to make room for themselves. Almost one-fifth of women in their fifties and sixties are divorced or separated. Increasingly women are initiating divorce, and regretting it less, even though they know it will be hard—emotionally, financially, and socially. It is a trial by fire. "Divorce reconfigures identity," writes Ashton Applewhite in *Cutting Loose: Why Women Who End Their Mar-*

riages Do So Well. "It requires that women come up with new ways of seeing themselves and road-test them under grueling circumstances." The challenge to a woman's ability to establish her own authority, and the enormity of the space she is carving out for herself by doing that can be overwhelming.

"The money stuff is the worst," several women told me. If ever the bag lady syndrome is out to get you, it is in these vulnerable circumstances. But once the divorce is over, most women emerge energized by the knowledge that they will never be so dependent—financially or otherwise—again. Lenore J. Weitzman, who conducted over 200 interviews for her landmark book *The Divorce Revolution,* found that "even the longer-married older housewives who suffer the greatest financial hardship after divorce (and who feel most economically deprived, most angry, and most 'cheated' by the divorce settlement) say they are 'personally' better off than they were during marriage . . . They also report improved self-esteem, more pride in their appearance and greater competence in all aspects of their lives."

It turns out they are also in better health. The conventional wisdom that marriage is good for you—the so-called marriage benefit—is being called into question. While it is true that married people, especially men, live longer than their unmarried counterparts, new studies are showing that a bad marriage is bad for one's health, particularly for women. Power, or lack of it, is an especially significant indicator. A fifteen-year Oregon study found, for example, that having unequal decision-making power was associated with higher health risk for women, but not for men (maybe because women don't have the other opportunities to exercise power that men traditionally do). Powerlessness is a major contributor to stress and depression. Tension and arguing can cause high blood pressure, reduce immune protection, and slow healing from injury and even from heart attacks. Dr. James Coyne, who studied the effects of marriage on recovery from congestive heart failure, told the *New York Times* (October 22, 2002), "Some of these people, if their spouses said, 'Breathe for the next half-hour,' they'd try to hold their breaths," he says. "It can get that stubborn in a bad marriage." The many women who say they initiated a divorce to save their lives may be literally right.

SAMANTHA'S STORY
"Until You Take Charge of Your Own Life, Things Don't Happen"

Samantha had spent over thirty years married to a raging alcoholic. She stayed with him for the children, and also because she believed him when he told her she would never be able to get along on her own. Then one day after their children had moved on, she sat down in her rocking chair, looked across at her husband, and told him it was over. "You will only fall on your face; you'll never be able to do it," was his response. "Just watch me!" was hers.

The catalyst for her action was a conversation with a woman she had worked with but knew only casually who turned out to be one of those right people who materialize at the right time. "She invited me out for coffee and said, 'I'm here to help you.' I had no idea what she meant. Then she said, 'I'm an alcoholic, and I'm going to help you break free of your relationship with him.'" Both women lived in a small town and Samantha's husband's drinking was pretty well known.

For two years, while the lawyers wrangled, she lived in the same house with the man she had come to hate. She barely slept because he kept the television going all night, while he lay passed out on the couch. There were also big financial problems. Her executive husband had been out of work for three years before the divorce proceedings began and, unbeknownst to her, had borrowed away almost his entire pension and built up IRS penalties. But she took courage from the conviction that "until you take charge of your own life, things don't happen."

She resumed her discarded profession in real estate and built up her skills. She also took up running; "Exercising got rid of that bad anger, and all of that stress," she says. There were times, though, when nothing could give her a boost. The day she discovered that a deal to sell the house they shared had fallen through for the second time, she remembered, "I just couldn't breathe. When I heard the news, I began to cry and couldn't stop. I kept thinking, I feel like I'm dead. I have no hope left inside me . . ."

Finally, she was able to move into a small house of her own, but it was two more years before the divorce became final. At that last meeting, she looked at her ex-husband-to-be and was overcome with sadness. "I finally let go of all that anger and hatred. He was so sad. He would never get his life together." But she had. "OK," she told herself, "my life starts here, now. I'm not going to live in the past."

"I don't feel fifty-six years old. I feel strong. I feel vital," she proudly reports today. "I've been able to support myself. I've fixed my home to my liking . . . and I have a nice man in my life." At first, though, she couldn't accept his attentions. "I wasn't ready and I was pretty tough on him—'get out of my face, who do you think you are, get out of my way.' Finally he said to me, 'I can see that you need some space. You are worth waiting for, so you take as much space as you need, and I will be waiting.'" And space *was* what she needed then, to consolidate her newfound authority.

One for One

Once a woman has taken charge of her life, the appeal of marrying again is not what it was the first time around. Now that space and authority are priorities. Mary had been divorced for twenty years. During that time she raised her kids, earned a professional degree, and moved from the midwest to Washington, D.C., where she knew exactly one person when she arrived. She had just bought a new fifties-style house that she loved and been appointed to a prestigious position in a professional organization, when she met a man who seemed on many levels to be the right match for her. He was retired, but expressed interest in her work. He enjoyed the out-of-doors as much as she did and had enough money to plan lovely vacations for both of them. He read widely and loved music. Their sex life was tender and satisfying. And he would sometimes take off for a couple of weeks on his boat, giving the relationship some precious breathing space.

Then he announced that he wanted Mary to marry him and sail with him around the world. A dream, yes, but *his* dream. Mary's plans were quite different. She was enlarging her business and was only halfway through remodeling her house. She was thriving in her new city—going to concerts, meeting new people every day, and enjoying her grandchildren. She tried to explain this to him, but he insisted that if they were to stay together, it would be at sea. "Don't make me choose between you and me," she told him, "because I will choose me." He did. She did. And although she misses the romance, she doesn't regret her decision.

Realistically, most women won't have to make the kind of hard choice Mary did. The ones I talked to were typically trying to make peace with the fact that the likelihood of bringing their newfound authority into an equitably shared space with a new partner was pretty small. They wouldn't have put it quite so bluntly, but they shared the estimation of sociologist Pepper Schwartz—who has written numerous popular books about sexual mores over the past thirty years—that a woman considering plighting her troth at this age, would most likely be taking on "if not a physical mess, an emotional mess." A man in his fifties or sixties, she elaborated in a down-and-dirty conversation we had, "may be very kind, he may be very bright, and have a lot of money—he may be all kinds of good things, but he will be less vital than her in a lot of ways. So, living with him is going to require a lot of stuff that she really doesn't want to do. And it will probably get worse. . . . For women who have got their act together—they're economically OK, they're physically OK, they've got vital lives—taking on something that will take away from that, as opposed to building it, is not a sound bet. And they don't make it. I think women are practical. I really do."

Every once in a while, though, all the pieces come together. Every once in a while, the new intimacy looks a lot like the old intimacy. When a dear friend got married for the first time at sixty-six, I couldn't figure out why a defiantly independent woman of experience and achievement was suddenly getting all mushy about love. Her response reminded me that nothing looks the same when you are not who you were, only older. She explained that after dozens of entanglements that didn't feel truly intimate, she was at a point in her life when romance—which has thrown many a woman's life off course when it comes (and goes) too early—felt just right. Why? Because once she had staked out her own territory, there was room left over for a little besottedness, a lot of companionship, and, after a long dry spell, some surprising sex.

Authority, Space—and Sex

We are the generation that was sexually defined by the pill and the 1973 *Roe v. Wade* Supreme Court decision legalizing abortion. What some called the sexual revolution was actually a reproductive rights revolution. For the first time in memory women were able to take control over their childbearing. The worldwide consequences are just beginning to be felt. To the astonishment of demographers, the population explosion they feared is turning into a population recession with major economic consequences for developed and less developed countries alike. For our generation, the personal consequence was equally historic: the separation of sex from reproduction. The parameters of our first adulthood were drawn by the empowerment of control over our bodies. The life-shaping event of having children or not and how many and when was no longer a fact of life but a choice that enabled us to plan our lives and invest in ourselves in ways our mothers could never have imagined.

As we now move into another unprecedented stage, the ability to separate reproduction from sex takes on new significance. While menopause may be the end of our reproductive life, it is not the end of our sex life. One of the major considerations in each woman's personal redefinition of intimacy is what part she wants sex to play. According to an AARP study reported by Claudia Dreifus in the organization's magazine (Winter 2002), sex qua sex does seem to be less of a priority for women over forty-five. They rank several other expressions of intimacy as more important, including "relationship with one's spouse, close ties with friends and family, spiritual well-being." Yet a solid majority also insists that a satisfying sex life is "important to their quality of life." In a way, the drop-off in sexual desire and the emergence of the Fuck You Fifties are a liberating combination. They make it possible to separate longing from lust, loneliness from solitude, and emotional servitude from commitment.

It should come as no surprise to the generation that has changed the rules so many times that we are in the process of doing so again. More women than ever are feeling more comfortable with their sexuality. In a *Newsweek* poll (2001), 30 percent of women between forty-five and sixty-five said they thought sex was better at their age than for younger people today, and another 41 percent said it was "about the same." Many are relieved to have some privacy and seduction time back after years on the fast track—the two-job/childrearing/ "having it all" lifestyle that was a mixed-blessing byproduct of our revolution. I was reminded of the sexual dry spell my friends and I went through back then (an early *Ms.* coverline read "How's Your Sex Life? Better / Worse / I forget") when I read about a spate of books—with titles like *I'm Not in the Mood* and *Okay, So I Don't Have a Headache*—that claimed to tell the truth about ways that tired and stressed out women of the next generation have found to avoid the added "to do" item of having sex. Evasions include feigning sleep and taking on all-night household projects like refinishing furniture or putting up preserves. Some things haven't changed.

The anecdotal impressions of our generation's sex life are soon to be bolstered by authoritative findings. The Kinsey Institute is engaged in the first major study of midlife sexuality. It includes research drawn from a wide range of disciplines and extensive in-depth interviewing, and the findings are likely to cause as much furor as those in the original Kinsey Report in 1953. An early conclusion is that older people are defying the stereotype of giving up on sex. Six out of ten people over forty-five who have partners continue to have sex once a week throughout their fifties—and at least once a month well into their seventies and eighties. Those who aren't, attribute the loss of desire to health problems (the single most pervasive turn-off) or simple lack of interest, though the researchers suspect the real problem is a lack of information about how their bodies are changing and what kind of satisfactions are still available.

The situation is complicated for women by two factors. One is access. As Marian E. Donn reported to the Kinsey Institute, "It may be difficult to maintain sexual interest and drive when the likelihood of finding an available and healthy partner diminishes." The second obstacle for those in a relationship, is familiar: "the emotional management business." Women, Donn observes, tend to function protectively. "When a partner is ill, unable to function sexually or is disinterested," she explains, "it is not unusual for women to say that sex is not important to them. They do not want to hurt the partner or make him feel inadequate." Another explanation is given by Dr. Lana L. Holstein who runs sexual awakening workshops for couples. Many women, she finds, are "midlife virgins" who "have had many sexual encounters, have birthed babies, but still have not claimed our sensual, sexual selves."

In general though, the sex we are having is more creative and uninhibited than has been considered seemly for people our age. The Kinsey researchers are uncovering a significant generation gap on the question of sexual experimentation. Women who grew up in the sixties and seventies report more interest in sex, more willingness to experiment, to engage in oral sex, to masturbate, to seek multiple partners, than the older women in the study. One Kinsey researcher asks, "What will be the effect on sexual attitudes and relationships in the future?" Another paper poses an even more provocative question about the prospects for present-day Second Adulthood women: "What resources—sexual, social and economic—can older women bring to the sexual marketplace that can overcome deeply ingrained cultural prejudice against their participation?" In other words, will our generation eroticize the image of an independent, energetic, adventuresome woman of experience beyond a handful of European movie stars—Simone Signoret, Anouk Aimee, Catherine Deneuve, Sophia Loren?

Many take-charge single women I talked to are finding out. They are lustily out there looking for the fifty-year-old version of Erica Jong's "zipless fuck" (described in her scandalous 1973 novel *Fear of Flying.*) They may be frustrated but they are not discouraged. Fran, who masturbates a couple of times a week for pleasure "and practice" thinks of her "sex drive like Nelson Rockefeller used to say about his presidential ambitions—he'd put them away, but if the occasion arose, he'd know exactly where to look for them."

But for nearly all of us, sex—however much or little we have—has become a form of self-expression. We are finally rejecting the high-stakes seduction game of artifice and manipulation in favor of a more forthright sense of our own desires. But how does one go about getting to know her "sexual self" at fifty, or sixty? Poet and counselor Ellen Bass, who for three years led sexual self-discovery workshops, noticed how bereft most women are of the kind of support from friends they get for exploring other areas of their lives. "If someone's having sex problems, a friend might say, 'Oh, that's too bad,' but we don't jump in the same way we do when they have other kinds of problems. We don't say 'OK, guys, what should we do about that?'" By the same token, we don't share our enthusiasm either. "It sounds funny when I say it," Bass adds, "but we act as though acknowledging that anyone has sex, in just a natural way, is really wild. Like if you're feeling really good one morning because you had good sex the night before, it's very rare that even with your closest friends, you'll say 'Oh, I feel great. I had great sex last night!'"

FRAN'S STORY
"My Sexual Responses Are as Strong as They Ever Were"

Fran, a fifty-nine-year-old divorced mother of two grown children, is the exception. She is particularly honest about her sexual needs and satisfactions, and the limitations of her circumstances. She is comfortable with her own sexuality and has made realistic decisions about its place in her Second Adulthood. Her forthright account reveals a woman in charge of her sex life:

"My libido is still definitely around, but it's much more selective these days. It's rarely stimulated by a visual—a good set of buns doesn't turn me on anymore. I now evaluate men my age (or a little younger) in terms of: would we be able to laugh afterward, and how comfortable would they be with me if they couldn't get it up—which very often they can't.

"Sex for a single woman tapers off. It was widely available in my thirties and forties but in my fifties there were only two men. Tim was a sensualist and a very good lover in terms of touching and foreplay, but not very satisfying because he couldn't manage to maintain an erection. Often I was very frustrated afterward, although the sleeping next to him and being held all night was nice.

"Jay is just the opposite, not at all a sensualist, but very vigorous (helped by Viagra, which he is quite open about). In some ways I'm not satisfied by that either. I wish he were more into touching and stroking, but one makes do. I often wonder whether it's worth it to try to teach him my ways—can an old dog really learn new tricks? He may be the last lover I have, and if that's true, maybe I should try to show him—he's certainly easy to talk (and email) to about it. But frankly I don't want to take the chance of alienating him—both on an emotional and sexual level.

"What I love about having Jay in my life is that I can anticipate that at some point whenever I see him I *am* going to have sex—the anticipation is almost as good as the act itself. And we can laugh—and we do—which makes it more than friction. Also there is something very wonderful about being with a long-time lover who's watched your body change and is okay with that. As a friend of mine said, 'there's a lot of artful draping going on.'

"Also with him, there's no question of where the relationship is going—we know we'll never be a permanent thing, yet both of us feel that if either fell in love with someone else, we'd really miss what we have. We are less interested in changing our lives at this point than we might have been. He's moved south recently, and we talk by email about when we'll see each other. Would I spend $200 to go visit him and get laid? Absolutely. And so would most women I know.

"The only thing I envy my married friends for—besides their greater economic security—is the availability (in theory, at least) of regular sex. I wish there was the kind of place I once read about in an English mystery novel—a club called 'A Certain Age' which was essentially a whorehouse for us dames. I would probably go. My sexual responses are as strong as they ever were, and I'm much more able to separate sex from love now than I once was."

New Frontiers of Intimacy

Other women find themselves willing and able to *join* sex with love in a way they hadn't considered before—with another woman. Ellen Bass, the poet, was once married and has a grown daughter, but for the past twenty years she has been living with a woman. In her sexuality workshops there were always a few midlife women who "have not felt that their relationships with men have been what they had hoped they would be. And a lot of women feel that they are more simpatico with women," she told me. "They feel that emotionally, and maybe this is the point at which they finally complete the picture. They feel that women are better listeners, more sympathetic, share better—play well with others—that they like those qualities in women. They like to be around women. They have liked sex with men, but the relationships were not in some ways as fulfilling as women's friendships were. In that situation they may then say, 'well, what the hell . . . yeah!' "

Pepper Schwartz has noticed the same willingness to go for it. "I think the impulse is helped by the fact that there was probably a lot of experimentation when the women were younger, in the late sixties and seventies, that took away some of the taboo. And even if we didn't explore those things earlier in our lives, even if we didn't activate them, some friend did, we read the stuff, we thought about it, it got into our fantasies . . . and for a life-long heterosexual it has the added advantage of being new. We are an animal that's titillated by the new, and in this case it has the kind of sweet blend of the thing that we're most comfortable with, which is our girlfriends, where we get the most emotional reward from, and then it's new—but not scary in the way it would be if we didn't like women so much."

A Circle of Friends

Divorced, widowed, and single women all say that their circle of friends is their primary source of support and trust, and most married women say the same thing. A study of well-being in the lives of one thousand working women by Nobel Laureate Dr. Daniel Kahneman, confirms, he told the *New York Times* (November 5, 2002), the "huge importance of friends. People are really happier with friends than they are with their families or their spouse or their child." A few good friends are as much a part of the new intimacy as our life partners and our sexual partners. They are the dinner partners of choice, as in my case. They are travel buddies, as in Vivi's annual forays to parts unknown. They are in our wills and on our buddy lists. We accompany each other to doctors' appointments and sit by one another's sickbeds. Even when we aren't in regular contact, we find it easy to pick up where we left off. Margo, the Peace Corps volunteer, discovered over the two years of only infrequent trips home that with good friends, "You don't drop stitches; you just put the knitting down."

I have one friend with whom I have worked out a shorthand way of touching base that is a model for me of shit-free, belly-laughing, empathic, smart, trusting intimacy. Our periodic phone calls begin with no salutation but a business-like "Are you waving or drowning?" The question is a reference to the lines in a Stevie Smith poem: "I was much further out than you thought/and not waving but drowning." We usually laugh—bitterly, happily, gratefully—at the question. Then, depending on the answer—which is always honest—the ensuing conversation can be tender or terse ("OK, just checking"). Even when I am drowning, she respects my *space* and my *authority*. She doesn't give me unsolicited advice about what to do, and I don't necessarily go into detail about what the problem is. What she does give me is the unequivocal message that she won't let me drown.

For many of us, such in-sync relationships are the working model for the new intimacy. We are most ourselves, most expressive of our authority, and most likely to feel taken seriously, in the truth-telling circle we create. The let-it-all-hang-out honesty we are getting good at is compounded in the safety of those circles. As a result, so is the intimacy. We are much more forthcoming about our failings and failures, more willing to seek and accept advice, less know-it-all about dispensing advice, and a lot less concerned with eliciting sympathy for its own sake.

It is in those friendship circles, too, that we experience the interdependence that takes the measure of the space each of us needs to get close to others. We listen, we ask, we intuit, and we forgive. The calibrations are refined by the gifts of gender—our empathic radar, our tend-and-befriend crisis-management style, our holistic approach to problem solving. Recent brain-imaging research has illuminated how much we benefit by working together. When women were studied playing a game in which they could choose cooperative or competitive strategies, the brain lit up most brightly when they chose cooperation—and only increased as the cooperation continued. (Men have yet to be tested for the same response.) According to a report on this study by Natalie Angier in the *New York Times*, the areas of the brain that lit up by cooperation were those that respond to "chocolate, pretty faces, money, cocaine, and a range of licit and illicit delights." All of which prompted psychologist Carol Gilligan to conclude that "sisterhood is pleasurable." It only becomes more so with age.

Recalibrating Friendships

While our friendships sustain us, they are still susceptible to the impact of our changing priorities. A tried and true circle of friends may need to be reconfigured; and new friends may answer new needs. British social psychologist Terri Apter found that one reason women go back to school—as some eight hundred thousand of us are doing—is "to meet other women." And one reason they were seeking new friends was that "Friends were often seen as necessary to growth—the 'groping together' was far more constructive than groping alone." Judy, who recently retired and relocated from the city to the rugged coast of Maine, puts great stock in the need for building a new support group to meet new challenges. "Reinventing yourself is about repackaging yourself," she said. "In the same way that women who are starting a business quickly form a network, we need to find advisors that can help us figure out what's next. Not all your current friends may be good at it."

Particularly as our circumstances change, the kind of support we need changes, too. Samantha had so much trouble extricating herself from a long and abusive marriage—"I was the enabler from hell!" Her lifesaver was the network of people who gravitated from the periphery of her life into her intimate circle. Because they had experienced what she was going through, they were able to give her the message she needed to hear: "You've got the power; and you are strong enough to do this."

Sometimes we have to renegotiate a friendship from both sides, to correct for a power imbalance. Carole Hyatt, who runs seminars for women executives, preaches the doctrine of networking, including among friends. "It's a skill," she says. "And there are people who don't want to network because it's giving something away. My mother didn't like introducing friends to each other, as though somehow they're going to take something away from her. It's like the recipe where you leave out the most important ingredient. There are two kinds of women," she has found, "those who give all the time—Lady Bountiful—but don't want to ask, and those who ask." She went on to describe an enlightening confrontation with a friend while they were sitting in a hot tub.

"She has called me in the last twenty years at least three times a week to request something. It's just her nature . . . and there we are sitting in the hot tub and she's spending thirty minutes doing this huge 'ask.' And I said, 'You know what?'— and I got very angry and made this splash!—'I have been hearing this conversation for the last twenty years, and you have never once offered me anything.' She looked at me dumbfounded. And she said, 'Carole, you never ask! You look like you have everything. I wouldn't even know where to begin giving to you, offering. I'd feel foolish.' And I said, 'Well, you run a business.' And she said, 'But you always seem to have clients. You always put on this wonderful front.' And I realized that I never did ask. That I have never 'lowered' myself to ask. That I was Lady Bountiful. And yet mysteriously I felt that she would offer. That everyone would offer. And the fact is that no one ever offers—unless you ask!" In all of her relationships, Carole is becoming aware that she needs to share the power.

Vivi was particularly aware of the bittersweet nature of the shifting demands of friendship. "There are friendships that evolve with you, that change and grow with you," she told me. "And there are friendships that change, where you feel you've moved beyond the constraints of the earlier configuration. But there's still tremendous love and warmth . . . and that's tricky." Making new friends is tricky, too, she says, "because you don't share that whole history, and you have to try to reconstruct your personal history." Vivi found Abigail through a common interest, singing in the choir of a synagogue Vivi had helped create (and ultimately broke away from). "She became a sort of mentor to me. . . . She's tough. And very bossy. But she's so correct, so right on." The friendship is now one of the most precious for both of them. "Abigail said one of the funniest things the other day. She said 'I usually don't make new friends unless someone dies.'"

Our friendships give us a model of intimacy in more ways than a framework of interdependence. "The only reward for aging," says sociologist Pepper Schwartz, "is a sense of some honest friendship with yourself, where you get to know yourself—you make peace with the things you are and you aren't." You see your life "filtered through a unique lens rather than a cultural one." In other words, intimacy begins at home. Before you can establish your authority, you need to know the sound of your own voice. Before you can take up space, you must be aware of your boundaries—and your reach. "The best cure for loneliness," wrote poet Marianne Moore, "is solitude."

CHAPTER EIGHT

Confronting Adversity

Time and trouble will tame an advanced young woman, but an advanced old woman is uncontrollable by any earthly force.

—Dorothy L. Sayers

I have always been captivated by the bumper sticker "My karma ran over my dogma." I see it as a sort of whimsical (that word again!) cousin to John Lennon's immortal "Life is what happens to you while you're busy making other plans." Both serve as a reminder that, no matter how many lists I make, how many emotional conflicts I negotiate, or how assiduously I research contingencies for a given action, life is going to seep into my fortress and crack the masonry. Somewhere in our struggle with the unknown of the Fertile Void most of us meet up with that insight, but it takes an act of will—or an act of fate—to put it into practice. Inner resources are what we find when we are called upon to cope with what we can't control.

Loss of control used to be the experience we dreaded most, and much of our energy went to holding on for dear life. Life is still scary, but now, in Second Adulthood, we are transferring our energies from managing our circumstances to taking responsibility for our lives—fears, failings, and all. A major agenda item of my Second Adulthood is to outgrow taking responsibility for everything. It has been pointed out to me by my family—not always with indulgence—that trying to micromanage life is a waste of energy and annoying to all concerned; and the record shows that my efforts have been only moderately successful. They are even less so as my children take on their own karmas. Nowadays, I literally bite my tongue against blurting out, "Did you remember to . . ." and for the first time in my life, I am trying *not* to overhear conversations that have the word "problem" in them. I'm experimenting with letting (human) nature take its course. As I let go of responsibility for smooth sailing for all in the waters around me, I find I am swimming with more abandon myself.

So far nothing cataclysmic has happened. My success rate is pretty much what it has always been. But in a few instances, the unanticipated outcome has been—well, unanticipated. At least once a week, what looks like a train wreck of fouled-up logistics miraculously falls into place—someone cancels (an option I never allowed myself when I was in charge), another unexpectedly offers to pick someone up, someone else comes up with a better (can you believe it!) plan. And at least once a month, some activity I thought wasn't worth the trouble of planning every last detail, right down to the route I would take to get there, finds its way into my schedule anyway and turns out to be fun.

Of course, I'm talking about the daily grind here, not the big stuff, but I'm hoping that I'm developing a more philosophical worldview—letting go of what doesn't really matter, experimenting with what seems to work, and getting on with whatever is next. If I don't, I fear I will waste the rest of my life hunkered down, futilely trying to fend off the evil eye. By controlling for every conceivable eventuality, the illogical logic goes, I will be able to outsmart the forces of catastrophe. The mellow frame of mind I am trying to cultivate combines an openness to what comes my way, good or bad, with the wisdom to make whatever judgment calls are in my best interest. And then move on.

That kind of easygoing autonomy is a new experience for women; just think of any corseted Edith Wharton character brought low by economic and social forces beyond her control. Until our generation, the area in which an ordinary woman was permitted to exercise control was limited to the four walls of her home, or more accurately, to the kitchen and the nursery. The rest of life happened *to* her; that's what made it so frightening. The freedom to take risks because you are confident you can deal with the consequences is what makes this stage of life exciting.

Mireille Guiliano, French-born CEO of the U.S.-based Clicquot Inc., has been taking professional risks for her entire career. "People are terrified of making a wrong choice," she says. She gets frightened, too, but when she faces a turning point in her life she hears her mother's voice asking, "What's the worst that could happen?" The irony, of course, is that the worst that can be anticipated isn't really so bad. So what, if you fail? So what, if it rains? So what, if they don't like you? And the worst that *does* happen usually hasn't been anticipated.

As I discovered when I took that step backward down a cliff and took control of my own gravity, with a firm grip on a safety rope, gaining control of our lives is also about relinquishing a foothold in the edifice designed to hold things together, but just as often held life at bay. The truth—especially hard for women whose mission it has been to hold everything together—is that taking charge isn't about control at all; it's about coping with the unexpected.

Nothing is more true for us now. While Second Adulthood is a time of delightful serendipity, it is also a time of great vulnerability. The big-ticket stress items that used to lurk in the shadows are now crouched on the horizon—loss of a job, loss of a loved one, a move, ill health, divorce, and rejection of all kinds. The unexpected is everywhere.

Mastery, Your Voice of Authority

While we certainly can't control for it, we are better equipped to withstand the evil eye than we have been at other stages in our lives. Second Adulthood brings what anthropologists call a sense of *mastery*. It is a gut feeling that you know what you are doing, even if it doesn't look that way to anyone else. Not all that long ago, women felt compelled to seek out and follow expert advice—from doctors, from magazines, from men. We believed that somewhere out there was an expert who would provide the right answer for us. Now we know that the experts are resources, but each of us has to be her own voice of authority.

Just talk to one of the growing number of women in their fifties initiating divorce. She knows she may end up lonelier than she is now; she knows she is exposing herself to financial risk; she knows that some of her acquaintances and, perhaps, even some of her children will be turned off; but she also knows—really *knows*—that the choice is right for her. She is the only expert worth listening to.

Anthropologists call this stubborn survivalist streak mastery, we call it life experience, and at least one humorist calls it a secret weapon. Soon after the military action in Afghanistan began, a sardonic suggestion surfaced anonymously on the Internet:

Women like us should be enlisted in the fight against terrorism because . . .
We've survived the water diet, the protein diet, the car-

bohydrate diet, and the grapefruit diet in gyms and saunas across America and never lost a pound. We can easily survive months in the hostile terrain of Afghanistan with no food at all! We've spent years tracking down our husbands or lovers in bars, hardware stores, or sporting events . . . finding bin Laden in some cave will be no problem.

Uniting all the warring tribes of Afghanistan in a new government? Oh, please . . . we've planned the seating arrangements for in-laws and extended families at Thanksgiving dinners for years . . . we understand tribal warfare.

Between us, we've divorced enough husbands to know every trick there is for how they hide, launder, or cover up bank accounts and money sources. We know how to find that money and we know how to seize it . . . with or without the government's help!

Let us go and fight. The Taliban hates women. Imagine their terror as we crawl like ants with hot-flashes over their godforsaken terrain.

A more academic description comes from David Gutmann, recently retired director of the Older Adult Program (Psychology) at Northwestern University. Anthropological research confirms a pattern of female independence and self-confidence emerging with age, and he writes: "Whereas adult males start from a grounding in Active Mastery and move toward Passive Mastery, women are first grounded in Passive Mastery, characterized by dependence on and even deference to the husband, but surge in later life toward Active Mastery, including autonomy from and even dominion over the husband. Across cultures, and with age, they seem to become more authoritative, more effective, and less willing to trade submission for security."

When poet and novelist May Sarton found herself confronted by a young woman unwilling to accept her contention that her sixties and seventies were the best years of her life, she responded with the best description of mastery I have found: "I am more myself than I have ever been. There is less conflict. I am happier, more balanced and (I heard myself say rather aggressively) 'more powerful.' I felt it was rather an odd word, 'powerful,' but I think it is true. It might have been more accurate to say, 'I am better able to use my powers.' I am surer of what my life is about, have less self-doubt to conquer."

The trajectory Guttman describes has been especially dramatic for our generation. Political and social forces have reinforced the cultural pattern to propel our emergence from dependence to independence. In the process, we have developed unique coping skills that will serve us well as we get deeper and deeper into the years that Bette Davis famously pronounced "not for sissies." As women told me of events that threw them off track, they revealed the inner resources that sustained and righted them, qualities that are emerging at this time in our lives as we need them.

No More Poor Me

The stories that follow dramatize the combination of pragmatism and conviction, mastery and willpower—shored up by a dedicated support group—that got these women through hard times. *Antisentimentality* is how I sum up the outlook that seems so out of character for this time of life. Given what I know about Second Adulthood, that should have been the giveaway, but it was only after listening to several women that I picked up on the no-nonsense matter-of-factness with which each recounted her experience. The subtext, as I read it, is that we've finally had it with romantic notions and operatic emotions. We don't need them any more; whatever reality is, we can take it.

One woman described her new pragmatism as a drive to "get over it." And move on. For her, "it" includes "old pain, shopworn expectations, talking things to death and bullshit in general . . ." Self-pity is out. Best selling self-help author Barbara Sher has little patience for those who "have been using hope to replace action." Her advice, too, is to get on with it. After all, she reminds those who are malingering in *It's Only Too Late if You Don't Start Now,* "sooner has passed and later has just showed up." An unexpected crisis can speed that process up.

MAXINE'S STORY
"There's Something About Having No Choice That Sets You Free"

Maxine would never have been considered a pragmatic, unsentimental woman. As a writer, and as a warm, exuberant wife and mother, she seemed to be riding on her bountiful emotions. She raised three generous, loving, citizens of the world with the man she had fallen madly in love with forty years earlier. Mark had been a devoted family man but a distant husband. His coldness hurt her, but she loved the warm and lively home they had created for their children, full of music and talk and good food and a deep religious commitment. Over all those years, Maxine had an illicit passion of sorts: the plays she kept writing—she couldn't help herself—which were sometimes produced in local theaters. Mark found her "hobby" troublesome, even though she also managed to contribute more than her share to the family income by other freelance writing.

Nevertheless, Maxine and Mark were heading into what they hoped would be calmer waters. They were making plans to spend more time on what they enjoyed doing together and on taking better physical care of themselves—just as soon as Mark returned from one last business trip. Then came the call: Mark had been taken off the plane disoriented and violent. When Maxine got to the emergency room an hour later, the doctors told her they suspected a stroke. Her children arrived and together they made the decision to let the doctors operate to relieve the pressure in Mark's brain. He was in a coma for six weeks. In the eighteen months since then, he has, in doctor lingo, "come back only about 20 percent."

This nightmare has taken Maxine on a year-long hegira from one medical facility to another—intensive care, good rehabilitation centers, terrible rehabilitation centers and, finally, a nursing home for stroke victims not expected to recover. Each transfer involved long drives to visit alternative options, and each facility was further from home. But that wasn't all. A second nightmare was fighting the insurance companies every step of the way, as well as the social workers and administrators who did their bidding. Maxine spent her days divided between Mark's bedside—massaging his feet, singing to him, begging him to wake up—and haggling with the system. She came away from this ordeal with the confidence that she could take anyone on, and the realization that she had accommodated too many bullies in the past. After a lifetime of winning over distant people with warmth, and meeting the objections of critics with reluctant changes in her work, "I don't want to have anything to do with people who frighten me or intimidate me," she proclaims.

Until this point in her life, Maxine had thought of herself as "a person who is pulled along by events"—in her case, some pretty traumatic events. Her father died when she was very young, and her sister came down with a degenerative disease when she was a teenager; as an adult she had withstood professional and marital disappointments; and in each case she had moved on. "There is a facelessness, a lack of choice in these events that makes the way quite clear, not because I chose it but because it chose me," she explains. But she is not fatalistic— quite the opposite. "There's something about having no choice that makes you free. Because the no-choice part anchors you, and everywhere you swim from that anchor *is* a choice."

As Mark stabilized, Maxine entered what she calls her "pre-widowhood." In a very methodical way she set about reorganizing her husband's business and dismantling the family home where they had raised their children. "I got rid of everything," she says, without sentiment, "except a few pieces of furniture that I had refinished for the kids. And the books." After she sold the house, everyone assumed she would move to New York City, where her friends and children were, and where the theater community that had sustained her flourished. But she didn't.

For one thing, she simply couldn't afford it. "I didn't have anywhere near enough money to live there. There wasn't even an option to be sentimental about." So she looked for a choice that was realistic. For months she had been commuting 250 miles to the facility near Boston where Mark was. Now, without fanfare or equivocation, she found an apartment there, one with a terrace big enough to house a miniature version of the garden she had cherished back home. "Boston was the best place to swim, given that I was anchored by financial necessity," she concludes.

Over the next several months, Maxine has contacted people in the area she had met or known in the past and, little by little, she is building a social life. Today, she goes to the theater and concerts and talks with her new friends about topics that bored Mark. She has gone into therapy to deal with the dark shadows of the past, she is working out and losing the weight that has plagued her, and she is writing. Plays. Novels. Whatever her imagination prompts. With more abandon than she ever imagined possible. "I have a whole new life," she says only somewhat sheepishly.

Once a month she takes care of business in New York and visits with her children and friends. Her children rotate weekend visits to their father. Maxine visits him every weekday and brings the homemade dishes he seems to enjoy. Some days he recognizes her and some days he doesn't. She continues to fight with doctors and medical services to get the care and attention she wants for the man she loved so much, but her attitude has changed. "I keep thinking of an episode of *Roseanne*," Maxine says. "She has taken a job sweeping up hair in a beauty parlor. She is dreading the job but it is the only one she could get and she is desperate, but it turned out to be fun because the people were fun." She feels that way about her situation. "I've come to think of the Mark part of my life like going back to school," she says. "I had to take this course in Mark being sick. It's a requirement. It's not a fun job. But the surrounding circumstances—the new city, the being alone, the being free, the new people—that makes it okay. That makes it doable. Even fun." Then, just for good measure, she slams the door on sentimental second thoughts. "I know it sounds cold, but the reality is that nothing will bring him back. And I can't give up my possibilities just to pretend it will."

Finding a Third Way

Maxine was able to cut right past the dream of *if only* to the real choices floating out there at the end of the circumstantial anchor chain. Sometimes, though, the choices are not clear, and the challenge is to look beyond the obvious. When confronted with what might appear to be a stone wall, going through it (fight) or retreating (flight) are not, as women continue to demonstrate, the only options. We have spent a lifetime preparing for finding other ways out. Because we "have not been permitted to focus on single goals but have tended to live with ambiguity and multiplicity," writes cultural anthropologist Mary Catherine Bateson, in *Composing a Life,* we have plenty of experience in coming up with innovative solutions to life's messiness and competing priorities.

A deceptively ordinary example of our style comes from a study of male and female commuters. The women, tracked to and from work, took elaborate detours, especially on the way home—to pick up ingredients for dinner, dry cleaning, glue for a school project, or a child at a friend's house. Men, on the other hand, made a beeline from point A to point B and back again. If there was an errand that couldn't wait until Saturday, they preferred to go out again later. Anthropologist Helen Fisher calls what we do *web thinking.* "Women think contextually, holistically," she explains, while men are more inclined to think in straight lines. An *either/or* zero-sum approach produces a limited set of outcomes. Our *both/and* way of thinking opens up infinite possibilities. This third way of inclusive problem solving is not a wimpy compromise between two alternatives, but a personally crafted approach that suits the moment, the circumstances, and the individual.

Both/and flexibility is the revelation of an essay "The Middle Way" by novelist Ellen Gilchrist (in the collection *The Bitch in the House*). Now sixty-nine, she only began writing in her forties, "after a struggle that included four marriages, three cesarean sections, an abortion, twenty-four years of psychotherapy, and lots of lovely men." Her commitment and success set off an increasingly debilitating family–work conflict. This is how she sized up the situation to herself: "I can let [family and work] be at war, with guilt as their nuclear weapon and mutually assured destruction as their aim, or I can let them nourish each other." The nourishment solution required some ingenuity as well as a bit of unsentimental toughness. She had to consider some options that seemed unthinkable, like leaving home, or impractical, like having her cake and eating some of it, too. She had to be unflinching in her assessments of how she would fit into each scenario.

Today she lives part of the time in the town where her husband and grown children live, and participates in their lives "as hard as I can . . . They don't have to ask for help. I see what is needed and I act. Then, when I have had enough of trying to control the lives of people just as willful and opinionated as I am, I drive back up to the Ozark Mountains and write books . . . and don't even think about my family unless they call me. If they need me I am here."

She says she has found peace. "I think I am happy," she concludes, "because I have quit trying to find happiness through other people . . . I derive happiness from the fact that my children and grandchildren are alive and breathing and that I am here to watch their lives unfold. Aside from that, it's up to me."

Keeping an Eye on the Half of the Glass That's Full

Attitude—how we interpret what is happening to us—is a choice. Not thinking like a victim is a crucial inner resource. So many of the stories I heard could have gone either way, toward despair or toward survival and growth. Certainly Maxine and Ellen Gilchrist could have fallen into either/or gloom.

Instead, they—like so many of the women I spoke to—opted to keep on keepin' on.

When I met Paula, she told me right off that she does not think of herself as a particularly happy person. "Things that maybe should make people very happy don't always make me very happy. I have a sort of cynical view of the world." Nevertheless, she has an attitude about hard times. "One thing that I realized is that when something major happened in my life— I met a man, he and I went out for fifteen years; it was a tumultuous relationship and then the relationship ended—I didn't crack up, or go crazy, or start drinking, or taking drugs. I thought, 'You know what? I'm going to reinvent myself!' I lost weight, I bought green contact lenses (God help me!), I moved into a new apartment, and I made it my business to get a promotion at work."

She was back on track when a few years later, she slipped on a drop of water in the kitchen and messed up her knee. When I talked to her she was homebound—and reinventing herself again. She was keeping her weight down by having diet meals delivered, and had taken up writing. "I hired myself a writing coach that I work with over the phone. I write a lot of stuff for kids. Right now I'm working on a story about plaid weasels." Although she had only a high school education, she kept up with on-the-job training and is proficient on the computer. This enables her to look for interesting topics to learn about, as well as to order all her household supplies online. She doesn't minimize this contribution of technology to her independence. Think of the isolation a woman in Paula's situation would have experienced in the past; no matter how self-sufficient she might have been when she was well, she would have been dependent on neighbors and family for everything from a carton of milk to the daily newspaper. Thanks to the Internet, Paula feels she has access to the best of both worlds.

Paula has no children of her own, but stays in close touch with her family and friends. "They call me for advice. If they are depressed, if they are sad . . . big time. It's not always about the joking . . . it's about 'well maybe your should try this' . . . I'm sort of good at doing that for other people. Not so great with myself." When she reads about how older women are invisible, she gets mad. "There are two types of human entities— the dead and the predead, so while you're waltzing from predead to dead, have a lot of kids in your life, laugh a lot (because life is ridiculous), have a lot of sex until the walls rattle, and have a good time." Ultimately, her reaction to negative thinking is "Shut up! Get on with your life!" No one would call her a Pollyanna, but, she seems to be saying about being predead, that *given the alternative* . . .

Of the six predictors of good old age that emerged from Dr. George Vaillant's study of adult development, two are particularly pertinent. The first is that bad events are not the unmitigated forces we sometimes think. "It is not the bad things that happen to us that doom us," he writes; "it is the good people who happen to us at any age that facilitate enjoyable old age." (It is intriguing to ask ourselves who those people have been in our own lives, and to watch for them in the life stories of others.) The second insight deals with how attitude affects the impact of events: "Objective good physical health was less important to successful aging than subjective good health. By this I mean that it is all right to be ill as long as you do not feel sick."

STEPHANY'S STORY
"I Will Not Be Bitter. I Will Not Be Bitter"

Stephany, who lives in a small midwestern city, was in her mid-forties when a series of depressing events struck that could have made her feel "sick." She had been a dutiful daughter of a woman who focused her life on her family, a supportive wife to a lawyer building a career, and a devoted mother of three. Then, in short order, all three outside sources of approval were withdrawn. When her mother died, it was a terrible blow. "I can remember thinking, 'who am I going to show my life to now?'" At the same time the last of her children entered full-day school, and her husband became increasingly buried in his work. Stephany felt very lonely, but she didn't allow herself to feel self-pity. She kept telling herself, "I will not be bitter. I will not be bitter."

She geared herself up to enroll in graduate school, no small effort. First she needed to get past one of her life's most crushing moments. The last time she had contemplated continuing her education, her mother was still alive and had encouraged her. "We'll pay for it," Stephany remembers her mother saying. But when she called home a few days later to say she was ready to sign up, her father answered. When she told him the cost, his reply was, "Well, who's going to pay for it?" "That was one of those times," recalls Stephany with pain, "when I couldn't speak. My whole body fell apart. My husband and I were already in debt. Obviously my mother had never talked to my father about it. When I recovered from that phone call—I don't know if I ever told my mother about it—graduate school just never came up again."

The financial situation was only somewhat better this time,

but the alternative—being bitter—was unacceptable. "Our house needed to be painted and at that time painting the house was less expensive than the cost of a master's degree, but we postponed it. It was exceedingly difficult for me to take that money from the family. I had this recurring dream that the house had been painted, but the paint job didn't take; it was blistering. Isn't that scary?" But her resolve was strong.

By the time she got her degree, three years later, she was separated from her husband. "I don't think they are related . . . Well, maybe they are." She suspects she precipitated the break. "I was feeling increasingly alone. I felt I was raising the kids alone. I was probably more demanding, and it was probably a lot of pressure for him living with me. At the same time, the more I did, the more he felt pushed away. And our kids were becoming teenagers. And that can be difficult, too." But the marital problems were more systemic. "He writes like a dream and he can make the most complicated idea understandable, but he's not comfortable around people. He has great difficulty in social interaction, which is what I thrive on."

"It was just a mismatch," says Stephany. "We both tried very hard." When the divorce came through two years later, it was a relief. There was no rancor, and she feels the financial arrangement was fair, but by leaving him, Stephany points out, "I quit a $100,000 a year job."

Being the only divorced woman in her inner circle of eight college friends only made Stephany more determined not to be bitter. She was hired part time to evaluate education programs: "I had been active in the League of Women Voters and the PTA. And I'd been a teacher. And I had this brand new Master's degree in educational administration." As her children became more independent, she took a full-time job and discovered that "most of the people there were maybe five years younger than

I, most of them weren't married, and they all had doctorates. So I started to think 'I've got to get a doctorate.' "

By then, at fifty-three, she was beginning to experience her mastery; she had picked up some momentum in her career and some confidence in her instincts. The same force—her interest in people—which propelled her out of her marriage fired her professional choice. "I enrolled in graduate school in psychology. I had no idea what psychology was about. If someone said that to me, I'd say that's no reason to study psychology, but I was just tremendously interested in people! There is no doubt in my mind that that was the most compelling interest I had." She had, in other words, found her passion. From then on, she was in charge of her life—come what may. The doctorate became the driving force. "I just had to finish this doctorate because then that would be mine and it couldn't be taken away," she remembers. "And if I screwed up it was my own fault."

Her choice closed off other options. She didn't allow herself to even think about meeting new men—there was just no time for that distraction. She also assumed a degree of economic anxiety in exchange for her tuition. "If I'd invested that money and taken some kind of other job, I would be much more secure financially now," she says. "But I remember talking to someone who worked in the mailroom; she had to be thirty years older than me. She said, 'Oh, Stephany, whenever a woman can do something to better herself, she should do it.' " Then, reflecting Dr. Vaillant's principle of positive influences, Stephany added thoughtfully, "You get this support in the most unexpected and unpredictable places, don't you?"

Although she now has a full-time position at a hospital, finances are still a problem. "Many of my friends have begun to retire. I can't possibly retire. As a result of decisions I've made. But I wouldn't want to retire. I love my work. I increasingly feel more sure of myself. I'm getting better at holding my own ground. The older I get, the more I'm able to say 'no, I don't agree with you on that,' even to very well-informed, well-educated, bright people. I'm more confident when I'm being challenged. . . . And, you know what? I don't feel bitter at all!"

A Safety Network

When attitude lags, and choices seem to be draining away, all is not lost if family, friends, colleagues, and the random right-people-at-the-right-time are holding a net. During Second Adulthood, a woman is reminded over and over that the community she built at work, the family she enlarged to embrace friends, the young women she mentored and the older ones she sought advice from, as well as those she instinctively befriended under stress—have become a support group larger than the sum of its parts. And we can count on yet another level of mastery and support from our inner circle. As the women of our generation have accumulated power, financial resources, influence, and expertise, we have been able to offer those resources to each other as well.

Every one of us who has made it through any downturn large or small has a story to tell about the endurance, generosity, and shared laughter of a community of friends. The following stories feature two very different kinds of community, the kind a woman builds for herself and the kind she plugs into.

TERI'S STORY
"You All Hang Out Just to Keep Each Other Honest"

"I come from a really dysfunctional, alcoholic family, that was violent," Teri begins. "I'm the oldest of five children, and the only girl—in a traditional Catholic family. So the burden of gender was . . . well, a burden. Being female felt like a curse. When I went into my hippie years, I believed in reincarnation, and I had this whole rationale that I must have been a terrible cad, a really bad *man,* in a past life to have wound up in this place." Looking back, she realizes, "I fought a lot of fights I didn't have to fight. The road was open before me, but I couldn't believe it . . . There were a lot of opportunities to step out and be one of those young shining stars, and I just didn't have the psychological make-up to step in." She also didn't have the backup of people who believed in her.

To escape home, Teri took a series of jobs that didn't pan out, and finally applied to the local community college. "I had screwed up so badly that I couldn't believe they would accept me, but I wrote them an essay about my sad little life. And they took me." At first she did well and got good grades, but she was also drinking heavily—"binge drinking was, like, a recreational activity back then"—and one night in her freshman year, she was raped in her apartment. "It was my roommate's brother, and I was too frightened to do anything, because the living room was full of drunken hockey players, and if I made a sound, I'd have the whole bunch of them in there . . ." She finished out the year but quit school and moved in with a "drunk who was also a drug addict." She got a job, at which she "promptly began an affair with my boss." And that's just the *first* twenty years.

But her survivor self—and an emerging passion for journal-ism—got her back to school. "What really got me back was that when I was there the first time I had joined the college pa-per and they really liked me. The school was pretty working class and everybody had to work, so it turned out there was no one to run the paper. Word got back to me that if I enrolled in school, there was a good chance I was going to get to run the paper. That was enough to get me back."

Her self-destructive self didn't stay out of the picture for long. "I think Duality is my middle name," she says wryly. She kept drinking and escalated her drugs. "I had already been through cocaine and getting myself off that," Teri recalls. "I'd already gotten myself off my favorite combo, phenobarbital and Scotch, and I had to get off Valium. Finally I had one of those deals where I kind of lost a day . . . when I came to, every cell in my body was screaming. I begged for God to take my life. And the sonofabitch didn't, so I went to my first AA meeting." That was the first time she reached out for help, and the group helped for a while. She finished college and was the class speaker at graduation.

Like a good girl, Teri got married soon after. Like a bad girl, she married a fellow alcoholic and pothead. When she left him seven years later, though, it was because he was belittling her survivor self's career plans. "The dynamic of the relationship was that he was passive–aggressive and I was aggressive–aggressive." When she finally decided to walk out, "it was almost like this reptilian brain thing. I left with $100 in my pocket and nothing else; I didn't take anything, because I felt so guilty about leaving. But I felt myself walking out the door feeling very light. Not happy—I felt broken in a lot of ways—but very light. Frightened, almost like I could blow away, and very light."

Determined to get her act together—entirely on her own—Teri moved south to a new city, got a new job, and finally acknowledged an attraction to women. But she chose "a very troubled young woman from a background far more harrowing than mine" and not likely to be much support. Then menopause hit "in a big way. It really changed everything. I don't think I look a million years old, but I look my age and I never did before. I was a pretty girl," she adds softly. "It's a comeuppance." It was as though everything had to fall apart before Teri could really begin over. "I really just broke. Every shred of identity that I had ever had was gone. I wasn't a married lady anymore, and I wasn't a journalist anymore, and I wasn't a heterosexual anymore. I wasn't even a Catholic anymore. So what the hell was I?"

Around that time she was working at a "make-do" job where she met an older gay man who helped guide her through the coming-out process. She describes him as "one of those angels who appears in your life, a magical, lovely person." The right person at the right time. "He caught on to me and embraced me and brought me into the gay community." It was the first time she felt she could let down some of her street-smart defenses. Soon she was hearing about "a gay AA clubhouse" which turned out to be in her neighborhood; she had walked passed it countless times. This time she took the *leap* that is the turning point in so many Second Adulthood stories. "One day I just went in. And lo and behold, it was a meditation meeting, a bunch of old hippies—which was right up my alley—a bunch of old gay hippies, and that is where I really sort of found myself." In that community she felt safe enough to stop fighting, look at her life, and begin the process of reassembling the fragments of her self.

One of those fragments is a childhood dream. "My whole Second Adulthood is about this performing life I have now. If I had had the wherewithal to defy my family, I would have been a performer. That's really my very first love." By day she works as a secretary, and she is mobilizing her newfound network to help her move into journalism. "Asking for help like this is a first for me," she admits. By night, within her recovery community, she is a jazz singer. "I do wacky stuff, too. I'll back somebody up on the ukulele; then I'll sing a jazz piece with a young kid that I sponsor. She plays the trumpet, so we drag her up on stage and make her play." Her group doesn't drink and hang around bars, but they do "love what the subculture has to offer" and make their own entertainment. "At the end of this week," Teri announces, "I will be performing in a very terrible talent show that involves a lot of boys in dresses . . ."

She is getting to know her core self among people who understand how intensely she has been resisting that confrontation. Teri's friends are in their twenties and in their sixties and come from a range of backgrounds and work experience, but they are all kindred spirits. "There's nothing to hide. You all hang out to keep each other honest, because that's when the disease comes in, when denial steps up." And they offer something very simple and precious. "Once I got involved in that community, I couldn't walk down the street without running into people that I knew. So there were always people to eat with, and have coffee with, and I have people who, when I start to isolate, call me up and say, 'Are you all right?' "

All in all, Teri says thoughtfully, she *is* all right. "I'm a whole lot more comfortable in my own skin now, and I have a lot more fun than I had as a young person." What's next? "There's a phrase from AA—'the wreckage of our past'—and I have a fair amount of wreckage that I need to attend to; some of that is damaged relationships, and a lot of it for me is money *mishigas,* but I'm working on it. I really like living alone, which is a problem when you are a lesbian. I'd like to find a lover who doesn't need to move in . . . I'd like to get to the point where I own a nice house and live by myself and write with impunity." A particularly poignant choice of words for a recovering self-punisher.

Finally, though, what makes Teri feel that she may have finally found herself is that she has a place not only in her own community but also in the human family as well. The young woman she is sponsoring is "someone who really requires a fair amount of time. But that was given to me when I really needed it, so I think it's the right thing for me to do, and it's really good for me . . . The stuff people that age do just blows my mind. But when you hear yourself saying the things that were said to you, it also keeps you sort of honest." There's one more factor. "I have moments of regret about not having children," she admits. "I made the right choice for myself, but it's hard not to feel sad sometimes. So it's nice to be useful to people who are the age my children would be."

KATHRYN'S STORY
"I Am a Survivor—Because of You!"

Jungian analyst Jean Shinoda Bolen calls cancer "the wisdom disease" because its relatively slow progress allows its victims to assess their lives—a high-intensity Fertile Void. Kathryn's support group was already in place when the disease hit. A sunny, energetic person, she had always watched out for others and made extended family a high priority. I met her through our children and always admired her place in their circle of friends: If she thought they should know what she thought was right, she would lay down the rules; if she thought she should know what they were up to, she would ask them straight out. Every one of those kids knew she would try to make things work out for them. When my son lost his ride to Woodstock II hours before leaving, his first response was a call to "Mrs. F," and she networked him a lift.

Kathryn was diagnosed with advanced breast cancer at fifty-two, just as her second child went off to college. A lifetime of sharing her energy and her ability to "make things work out" with others had produced a wide circle of concerned friends and colleagues who wanted to do whatever they could for her now. That she benefited mightily from this support is clear from the regular e-mails she circulated to her inner circle over the next eighteen months. The excerpts that follow are testimony to her inner resources—her honesty and humor, her mastery and pragmatism, her I'm-ill-but-not-sick attitude—and to the vital role played by the loving support group that her own generosity of spirit had bound to her.

8/13. I had the weekend to digest Friday's info and now realize i am VERY lucky to not have this spread to other organs. [My doctor] said it means my immune system is really good to fight off such a large tumor. so I am hopeful, still scared, but will gather info, digest it and choose the treatment I feel is right for me . . .

PS my current therapy is to FEED MY SPIRIT, therefore:
- Tomorrow Madame Tussauds Museum and The Lion King
- I'm driving to visit [my daughter who is a camp counselor] at camp with my niece and THE BABY . . . that should be GREAT therapy!!!
- Thurs. I have an appt. in the city for my wigs.

9/6 (I AM HIGHLY AT RISK FOR CANCER TO RETURN AT A DIFFERENT SITE!). Therefore, aggressive treatment is justifiable. I will be on a very aggressive form of chemo . . . I will be infused day 1 and again on day 8, then have two weeks off and repeat the cycle. This will continue for 6 MONTHS! After 6 months of that, I will then get 5 treatments every 3 weeks of Taxol, another drug. After that I will have nipple reconstruction, and a month later, I will have 5–6 weeks of radiation. Sounds like this will take about a year!

I am totally freaked out, but will relax this weekend to

gather my inner strength. I know mentally that I must be strong, positive and be happy that there is treatment available for my breast cancer—all good things, but emotionally I'm a wreck . . . scared of the unknown . . . So hard for someone like me who likes to be "in control." Likes to plan and write down in my appointment book all my "doings" (I know, you're laughin girls . . .)

5/12. I have had 13 radiation treatments, with 20 more to go. I am often tired, but thankful for the loving support of my family and friends. I AM A SURVIVOR!!

Today was Mother's Day. . . . As we sat down for lunch I thanked Elliot for making me a Mother. A most wonderful, exciting, exhausting, and exhilarating job.

He said, 'Well, if you could do it over again would you marry me?' I said 'Of course!' And he said 'Good, cuz that's why [our rabbi and his wife] are coming at 4 o'clock to marry us in the Jewish tradition.' I've always felt bad about not being married in a religious ceremony (we were married by a Justice of the Peace) . . . I wore the same hat I wore when we were first married. I actually knew right where it was !!! So, for me it's been a glorious day.

6/17. It's been almost a year since I found the mass in the breast. It has been an incredible journey. A journey which has been life-altering.

I want to thank you all for your love and support. Whether you sat with my family during my operation, took me to treatments, held my hand while I was scared and throwing up, made meals for my family, made homemade soup for me, when it was the only thing I could keep down, sent me flowers, wrote a note, called to check up on my progress, or just kept me in your prayers . . .

So to all of you, I thank you: I AM NOW A SUR-
VIVOR because of you!

- To my husband, who has been my coach and anchor.
  Who saw me at my worst and still said I was beautiful . . . I am a survivor and will continue to be because
  of him. He is my reason to live!
- To [my children] who I'm sure were frightened and
  didn't know what to do, but always seemed to do the
  "right and caring" thing. They are my reason to live!
- To my sister who took her two week vacation to nurse
  me post-surgery, who bathed me, washed my hair
  (when I had hair), cooked for my family and just was
  there for me. She is my reason to live!
- To my business partner who told me to forget the business and take care of my health, that should be my #1
  priority (even when I fought to stay working). He is my
  reason to live!
- To all my friends; you were instrumental in my journey,
  you helped me with research, got me fast doctor appointments, educated me on the latest treatment proto-
  cols, made phone calls for me, you were there to
  comfort me, make tea for me, bring me goodies, drove
  me to get my head shaved and pick out my wigs, took
  me to treatments . . . laughed at how I tried to pencil in
  my eyebrows when I had none, and who now tell me
  that I look good with only 1 inch of silver!!! hair. You
  are all my reason to live!

My journey is not over, I know. But the treatments are. I
am a Survivor, I feel, for having survived the treatments.
They were long, painful, but I feel thankful that with today's
research, I am the lucky one . . . I am grateful that I have
lived a great life . . .

7/23. Tomorrow is one year since my surgery. A year that has changed me for the better. A year that has made me more tolerant, thankful and content. A year that validates for me just how precious time spent with family and friends can be.

11/22. I'm baaaack, so to speak. I've just returned from my oncologist. . . . All my tests are normal, my cholesterol is 174!!!! and I'm in the lowest risk group for heart disease (a worry since both my parents died from heart disease!)

So Happy Thanksgiving . . . there will be no more "updates" cuz now I am putting this experience behind me and moving forward . . .

TO LIFE!!!!!

To Life, Indeed!

When adversity struck, the women in each of these stories took responsibility for the hand they were dealt and moved on from there. They didn't waste time and energy trying to gain control over what life was dishing out or in feeling sorry for themselves. Instead, they found the resources they needed to keep them going within themselves and in their lives.

Buffeted by circumstances, they managed to zero in on What Matters. They developed expertise—mastery—by improvising and figuring out What Works. And they got through it—as they were changed by it. Today each one is not who she was, but she is stronger. And even more ready, willing, and able to meet What's Next?

I am not sure I could be as upbeat as Kathryn or as resilient as Teri or as tough-minded as Ellen Gilchrist or as conscientious and energetic as Maxine or as patiently determined as

Stephany. Or as totally lacking in self-pity as each of them. But when my bad karma runs me down, as I know it will with increasing frequency in my Second Adulthood, I will have their examples—and my own circle of beloved friends and family—to call upon.

Moving On to What's Next:
Making Peace and Taking Charge

CHAPTER NINE

Health, Beauty, and What You Cannot Change

*. . . I was never a pre-Raphaelite beauty
nor anything but pretty enough to satisfy
men who need to be seen with a passable woman.
But now that I am in love with a place
which doesn't care how I look, or if I'm happy,
happy is how I look, and that's all.*

—Fleur Adcock, "Weathering"

As a Christmas gift to his clients, my physical trainer had T-shirts printed up with his name on the front and an inspirational message on the back. He is an encouraging, personal-best kind of taskmaster, so I was totally unprepared for his choice of a motto: "No one trains for second place." As a matter of fact, I didn't grasp the meaning at first; the notion of competition is so alien to my fitness experience. For most of the women I know, working out is part of a larger personal-best goal: well-being. That includes paying more attention to our one and only body, accepting its accruing limitations, and working around, not against them.

All of Second Adulthood is about Making Peace and Taking Charge. Nowhere is that more explicit than in the area of health and well-being. Attending to our aging bodies calls upon whatever expertise, confidence, and energy—as well as the wisdom to let go when prudent—we acquire along the journey. Managing our physical well-being also calls for regular exercise of our most full-throated *no* in response to conventional wisdom that is wrong and expert advice that doesn't apply to a given woman's body. Every woman has to become as educated about her body and the options medical science is coming up with as she is about her finances. If she neglects either one—becoming, in the words of the country song, "Cleopatra, Queen of Denial," Second Adulthood will be wasted on her.

Our approach to health care is already much more aggressive than back when, for example, male gynecologists were performing hysterectomies right and left, and women were acquiescing to their authority. Today, we question what is presented as inevitable. We research our complaints and the diagnoses we are given, we share homeopathic wisdom, we accompany each other to second and third opinions. And we workout. *Fit* has superseded *fat* on the self-esteem radar screen. As one woman told me, "I used to weigh myself twice a day; now it's hardly twice a month. I just love being able to put my own suitcase in the overhead rack."

We have taken to heart the fact that thirty to forty minutes of exercise a day reduces stress, cholesterol, and blood pressure, preserves bones, and heightens mood and energy. As one woman, who swims a mile and a half twice a week, said, "You think about things that might worry you, but you're not as worried because you are physically busy. . . . You worry in a different way." She does yoga too. "You almost can't worry," she says, "because of the breathing and because the difficulty of some of the positions engages you . . . You get to the point where you zone out. To me that's the best. I think that gives me a lot of energy."

Some women, like Joanne, the late-blooming free-spirit dancer, have found that taking on a new physical challenge propels them across personal frontiers, too. Fran, whose sedentary lifestyle left her with a, shall we say, buoyant body type, took up scuba diving at forty-eight and plunged right into her Second Adulthood. "It expanded my vision of who I could be and what I could do. It gave me the confidence to take other risks like moving across the country and going back to college and falling in love again."

Working out is the easy part of taking care of our bodies. It is under our control, a matter of willpower. Almost everything else—from figuring out how seriously to take certain aches and pains, to making major medical decisions—is a matter of research, judgment, and (given the current state of the health-care system) sheer grit. Moreover, new and revised information can change the picture from one day to the next. Perhaps the best advice is to manage our well-being in accordance with the guidelines found in the ancient prayer: "Lord, give me the strength to change what I can change, the courage to accept what I cannot change, and the wisdom to know the difference."

"What I Cannot Change"

There are plenty of annoying and debilitating physical changes that begin taking place around fifty, in addition to those specifically associated with menopause. They include:

- Thinning hair (all over)
- Weight gain (on average about fifteen pounds), mainly in the middle
- A need for reading glasses
- Memory loss

- A decline in the ability to multitask with agility
- Bone loss (up to two inches in height over thirty post-menopausal years)
- Loss of elasticity in the skin
- Bladder problems
- Changes in sleep patterns
- Adjustments in the body's thermostat (sweat glands may disappear, making you more sensitive to overheating; circulation slows down, making you more sensitive to cold)

"To Change What I Can"

Certain conditions are more inevitable for some of us than for others, depending on our personal histories:

- Aches and pains
- Depression and anxiety
- Loss of libido and vaginal dryness
- "Widow's hump"
- High levels of stress
- Arthritic joints

"And the Wisdom to Know . . ." About Major Health Risks, New Treatments, and the Peculiarities of My Own Body

These potential sources of catastrophe require constant vigilance:

- Skin cancer
- Breast cancer

- Lung cancer (the most common cancer-related cause of death among women—and rising)
- Hypertension (cardiovascular disease is the number one cause of death and disability among American women)
- Alzheimer's disease
- Misuse of medications (including herbal ones)
- HIV/AIDS (yes, AIDS!)

Making Peace with What I Cannot Change

It takes all the mellowness we can muster to accept some of the humbling surprises our bodies present us with. We know it shouldn't matter—it is how we live, not how we look, that is important. As French journalist Françoise Giroud, who wrote her last column just days before she died at 86, put it: "Youth is short. It is life that is long." But it *does* matter. We have days when, as my friend Kate moans, we feel "old and fat and stupid." On those days we need all the help we can get. Luckily, we bring from our first adulthood championship-level expertise in two powerful coping tactics: truth-telling, and humor. Each is taken to new heights in our brazen and no-nonsense fifties and sixties.

In the truth-telling department, I know more than I ever expected—or in some cases wanted—to know about my friends' vaginal dryness and sagging breasts, backaches and sneeze leaks. One of the last taboos was broken in Letty Cottin Pogrebin's book *Getting Over Getting Older,* which describes the graying and thinning of pubic hair. Hundreds of women who read the book told her how liberating it was—as always—to find they were not alone in this secret shame when, as Pogrebin puts it, "the pubic went public."

Recently, actress Jamie Lee Curtis took truth-telling to a professionally risky level for a woman whose athleticism and perfect silhouette has been her stock in trade: she unveiled her forty-three-year-old body in the pages of *More* magazine without makeup and flattering lighting and other tricks used to "show her at her best." Instead, she just stood there in front of the camera wearing worn workout clothes, with her waistline forming a small life preserver above her Lycra shorts and dimpled thighs. Referring to her glamorous, youthful image, Curtis says, "It's such a fraud. And I'm the one perpetuating it." For the scores of women who responded with gratitude, that photograph was a moment of truth. It was comparable to when Gloria Steinem rejected the option of hiding her age behind her beauty and told the world, "This is what forty"—and subsequently fifty and sixty and, incredibly, seventy—"looks like."

Knowing what fifty or sixty looks like when people who could get away with fudging ten years admit their age goes a long way toward demystifying the aging process. But knowing how old other people are doesn't answer the haunting question: "How old do *I* look?" I am particularly sensitive to this question, because, since my children are still young, I am often thrown in with a younger generation than my contemporaries who are becoming grandparents. Those of us who waited to have children tell each other that having them now "keeps us young." That is true, if only to the extent that we don't have the luxury of time to brood about aging. But when I see younger parents trying to figure out how to relate to me, and when a teacher young enough to be my daughter struggles to impress me with her maturity, I know I am confusing others, too.

My body gives more mixed messages. I have always been strong—I had no trouble with overhead suitcase racks—but I was never really physically fit. Whenever I went out to play softball with my colleagues or to play a rare game of tennis, I got winded easily and usually pulled a muscle. The irony is that back then I was firm on the outside and flabby on the inside; now I look flabby, but I am clinically more fit than ever.

I play age games with myself. I tell myself I am reaching for the handrail more often because the subway stairs are less well lit. I convince myself that my wrinkles are still dewy, while those on the old lady over there are crepey. I tout elasticized waistbands for women of all ages. There have been countless occasions when I had to restrain myself from going up to a perfect stranger who I assessed to be a contemporary and asking her age. What holds me back, despite my new audacity, is the realization that I don't really want to know. Instead, I now try to define my age in a way that doesn't depend on what I look like to the person-in-the-street but on what I feel like to the person inside. When put through the Letting Go and Saying No (and yes) filter, here is *me*—at least for now:

- Old enough to know better, young enough to take a risk
- Old enough to keep my cool about most things, too old to be totally cool
- Too old to be taken seriously in some circles, young enough to get mad about it—and even get even
- Old enough to set my goal weight at the point I used to start dieting, young enough to think I can get there
- Old enough to look foolish doing some things, foolish enough to laugh at jokes about "old ladies"

Truth telling combines with laughter to the bad-news/good-news beat of the making peace process. And the older we get, the more material for humor we have. Sometimes it is light-hearted. For example, a friend and I devised an alternative for the phrase *senior moment*. The new term grew out of my constant frustration at being unable to retrieve the name for a spectacular flowering tree in my living room. Everyone asks what it is, and each time I have to run through the alphabet, more than once, to finally come up with "hibiscus." When I told this to my friend, we agreed that from then on we would refer to it as a "hibiscus moment" instead of the other kind. There is a sweetness to the phrase that takes the sting out of memory lapse. Poet Ellen Bass has another phrase for those humiliating moments. Standing at the counter of a store, suddenly unable to remember her social security number, she recognizes what she calls "an *I Love Lucy* episode of the mind." In the same vein, Michela Gallagher, a neuroscientist studying the aging brain, deadpanned to an audience of fellow researchers, "It is clear that many people would benefit from something like bifocals for the mind."

Most of the time, however, the humor is more bitter than sweet. Though still pretty funny. I have files full of potshots that have been circulated on the Internet. Here is one example:

Subj: what a difference 30 years makes

1972: Moving to California because it's cool
2002: Moving to California because it's warm

1972: Growing pot
2002: Growing a pot belly

1972: Trying to look like Marlon Brando or Liz Taylor
2002: Trying NOT to look like Marlon Brando or Liz Taylor

1972: Acid Rock
2002: Acid Reflux

1972: Going to a new, hip joint
2002: Receiving a new hip joint

1972: Whatever
2002: Depends

You get the idea.

To Change What I Can Change—Taking Charge

One-size-fits-all is as invalid in health management as it is in muumuus. Osteoporosis, for example, can be treated from several directions—medication, exercise, diet—with a wide range of success, depending on the rest of a woman's medical picture. The same goes for arthritis. Depression and loss of sexual interest can be the result of any combination of changes in the body or psyche. Treatment may involve coordination of several specialties. The point is not to take no for an answer until you have checked it out to your satisfaction. Even then, it's worth revisiting the evaluation process periodically.

The most serious threat to the management of our well-being is the dismissive power of ageism. Buying into a negative stereotype about our age group makes it more likely that a woman will accept as permanent what is very possible to change about her personal aging process. "Aging is about adult development," Dr. George Vaillant, author of *Aging Well,* told a Harvard Club audience, "not unrefrigerated fish!" He went on to argue that the decay model is literally bad for our health. Not only because the medical profession is not paying enough attention to the process of aging, but because individuals with a fatalistic mindset will not be proactive about their well-being.

Ageism is everywhere—even in our own hearts. Sometimes I find it hard to contain my impatience with a woman who may be only a few years older than I am fumbling for her credit card. I know I have discounted an opinion proffered by a woman with white hair and a quavering voice. We are talking the talk about exuberant aging—with good reason—but we don't always walk the walk. Having asserted our worth against the prevailing contempt for women throughout our first adulthood with such success, we face at least as big a challenge in respect to the image of the older woman.

That is particularly hard to do when the only image of our age group is in our friends' faces and never on the billboards or in the magazine ads that stare back at us. An older woman is not a pretty sight to those who sell beauty. Women over forty-five spend two-thirds more on beauty products than women aged eighteen to thirty-five, but cosmetics are advertised as though we didn't exist. A walk-the-plank mentality has cut short the careers of older models. Isabella Rossellini was dismissed as the spokesperson for Lancome cosmetics in 1995, soon after she turned forty, not because she was no longer beautiful, but because focus groups reportedly convinced the marketers that older women want to identify with youth. If true, their contempt is another disheartening example of what early feminists dubbed "horizontal hostility"—rejecting the person who is like you because it is too frightening to fight the powers that are putting you both down.

Women can combat that contempt and take charge of changing what they can change. One way we do it is by paying attention to our appearance or, as a friend of mine who cherishes antique words, likes to refer to it, our "grooming." But to get it right, we still have to face some facts. The way that model Lauren Hutton, who is sixty, reevaluated her looks is a particularly instructive case in point; it is a Second Adulthood story about reinventing her business as well as her appearance. She began our interview with a little first adulthood background. After a modeling career that began in 1974 and fizzled in the early nineties, and after a disastrous relationship with a man who managed and lost some $13 million of her money, she pulled up her socks, learned what she needed to know about money, business, and her face, and started all over again.

That brought about a close encounter with her then fifty-six-year-old self as it appeared in photographs. "I looked like a thirty-years-older alcoholic monster," she told me. Since she had always done her own make-up, she decided she was the best person to analyze and remedy the situation. First she had to accept a few things. With aging, her skin had lost collagen and water, making it dryer and more transparent. And she had put on almost twenty pounds after a lifetime of thinness. ("This was great for filling out the wrinkles, though," she added.) Indeed, "everything had moved!" The shadows she had lived with and concealed with makeup had shifted. She realized that, for example, as the skin at the bridge of the nose becomes thin, the cartilage underneath shows through, making the eyes look closer together. This face would require a whole new approach.

For one thing, the "girl" makeup that had been used in the "ugly" photos had too much pigment. "Since less blood is circulating in the skin, everything fades. If you put on the same makeup you used in your twenties you look garish, like a tart." So she set out to develop her own line of age-appropriate cosmetics and application techniques called Lauren Hutton's Good Stuff and marketed it on the Internet. Today, her modeling career is thriving and, like thousands of other women-owned businesses that are quietly changing the economy, so is her business.

Having experienced her own renaissance, she is a big believer in Second Adulthood woman power. "We're part of this gigantic crest, this extraordinary generation of women who haven't hit the shore yet," she proclaims. "Our wave is at its peak, and it's going to roll for quite a while. And we're going to have this enormous wall of power when we hit."

Makeup is one thing, and most of us take advantage of what it can do. Plastic surgery is another story, one we are more conflicted about. Judi Dench, sixty-nine, the great British actress is a poster girl of sorts for the natural look. Her beauty, her sly wit, her sexiness—*and* her wattles—add up to a model of authenticity. The alternative, in the words of Susan Sarandon, fifty-eight, another actress whose face looks defiantly lived in, is to look like a "female impersonator version of myself." For these two women, the choice has direct professional consequences, but for many ordinary women, looking younger has complex personal meanings. Cosmetic surgery is a $7.5 billion business. (Botox injections, the fastest growing category of medical beauty treatments, brought in a whopping $634 million in 2002.) "I want to look as young as I feel" is a common explanation, or "I don't want to look so tired" or "I just hate the way I look and I want to *like* the way I look."

Beyond the fact that plastic surgery can be dangerous as well as prohibitively expensive, my own criterion is to do only what can be done once and for all, and nothing that involves invasive surgery (like liposuction). Several years ago, I decided to have the one-time procedure of removing the puffy bags under my eyes, and I am happy with the result; I feel that my less tired-looking face is more expressive of my well-being. But I can't bear the idea of getting injections that would paralyze my forehead on a regular basis and watching myself age over and over again in the time in between, even though I am envious of the worry-free look. I marvel with my five regular dinner partners over the pileup of accordion pleats around our necks, but if any one of them decided to go for a face-lift, I would support her.

It's hard to sort out our motives. Are we buying into the youth culture or still trying to please men—pressures that countervail the inner confidence we are feeling in so many other areas? Or are we exercising the precious option of personal choice, emboldened by a new sense of confidence and self-determination? Only one person can know for sure. And she is in the process of finding out.

If We're Not Old Ladies, We Are Most Definitely Not Small Men

Even more detrimental to our health than the assumptions about the decline of old age and the dismissive attitude toward old ladies are the assumptions about how women's bodies work. The idea has been that, for all intents and purposes, we are merely "small men." Not only *can* we change our attitude, but we *must* insist the medical community change theirs, too, because such presumptions directly affect the treatment women are offered. Until very recently, medical research that did not have to do with the reproductive organs was performed on male subjects and then extrapolated for women by adjusting for weight. This protocol resulted in a body of knowledge that was often misguided. The most well-known example is how doctors were taught to recognize symptoms of a heart attack: shooting pains, usually down the left arm, shortness of breath, the sensation of a heavy weight over the chest area. It turns out that those symptoms hold true for most men, but women often present a very different pattern: light-headedness, profuse sweating, indigestion-like discomfort, "feeling funny." Those much less dramatic complaints were regularly dismissed as insignificant, often with fatal consequences.

Dr. Marianne J. Legato, one of the first to point out this life-saving difference between male and female symptoms, has followed up with a wide-ranging report on the consequences of practicing "small men" medicine. "As we compare men and women," she writes in *Eve's Rib: The New Science of Gender-Specific Medicine and How It Can Save Your Life,* "we are finding that in every system of the body, from the very hairs of our heads to the way our hearts beat, there are significant and unique sex-based differences in human physiology." When the genders are studied independently, dramatic distinctions emerge that are only beginning to be factored into diagnosis and treatment.

There are some conditions that no one would have discovered in small men. One of Dr. Lagato's examples explained a minor but persistent ache at the base of my thumb. The pain, I learned, is the result of years of wear on the distinctive configuration of bones in a woman's hand. Other conditions produce dramatically different responses in the male and female body. And certain diseases show distinctive patterns *among* women, which—for obvious reasons—do not show up in the small men research. For example, diabetic women are less likely than non-diabetic women to suffer from osteoporosis but are four to six times more at risk for coronary artery disease. It also helps to know that women feel pain more intensely than men do and are "more likely to have pain at a distant site from the part of the body with the problem. (This is called *referred* pain.)"

The gender factor expands the possibilities for diagnosis and treatment, particularly in the much debated and little-understood realm of body/mind interaction. And more particularly in the understanding of two conditions—depression and stress—that can affect the decisions we make in Second Adulthood.

What's All in Your Mind—and Your Brain

Men produce 52 percent more serotonin, which prevents depression, than women do. Such findings about brain chemistry combine with discrepancies in life experience—success, like recognition for one's work, is known to increase serotonin—to suggest different treatments for women. Since women often get less recognition than they deserve for much of what they do, it is intriguing to prescribe, as Dr. Legato suggests, therapies that enhance "feelings of independence and control." Recognizing and managing depression is an ongoing concern, because it is easy to confuse depression with "making peace with reality" and to turn the wholesome process of "letting go" into the morbid defeatism of "giving up."

Stress, a major cause of wear and tear on our systems, is similarly gender-influenced. Unrelenting stress lowers immune levels, burns out the digestive system, the circulatory system, and the nervous system, and throws off all our body rhythms. It is the antithesis of wellness. But the inner workings of a stressed-out female body hold some mysteries. Until recently stress was assumed to release the fight-or-flight pattern of chemical changes in all humans. We now know that men respond this way while women exhibit a tend-and-befriend response (see Chapter One) and experience a dramatic reduction in stress-related symptoms when they receive the support of other women. It is interesting to speculate about what results a therapist treating a woman for stress might get by focusing as much on the quality of her patient's support network as on, say, her job or her marriage.

Before any of us accepts a complaint as something *I can't change,* we need to make sure that what is known about the condition is based on research on a physiology like ours. For many women that means developing expertise by tapping into (trustworthy!) Internet resources, in addition to consulting the old reliable network of informed friends, women's magazines, and books. Then we need to make sure that whatever scientific information we assemble is matched by an equally well-informed dossier on the idiosyncrasies of our own bodies. This, in turn, calls for a professional team of specialists for some things, generalists for others, and advisers on matters that are not clinical—including learning to pick up the messages from within.

The Wisdom to Know . . . That Medical Knowledge Is Changing Every Day— and so Is My Body

For any woman who is not eager to make a career of keeping ahead of the rumors and misinformation, the mixed-blessing department is particularly maddening. Every day we hear about research findings that have an on-the-one-hand-and-on-the-other-hand message. Not long ago it was reported that the assiduous application of sunscreen to protect against skin cancer also blocks out crucial amounts of vitamin D, which we get from casual exposure to the sun. The remedy for a sunscreen-induced vitamin D deficiency is short periods of unprotected exposure—but how long is "short?" Never has it been so important to tailor our health regimen to our very personal conditions and circumstances. "In consultation with a physician," we dutifully add, knowing full well that we can't stop there.

Sometimes the most conscientious doctor is uninformed or is reluctant to broach a particularly touchy subject. How many of us, for example, have been asked by our doctors if we are practicing safe sex? Given the fact that our age group includes one of the fastest growing populations of HIV/AIDS infection (women in their forties, particularly in the African-American community, but among older women as well), we should all be talking about it. There are several explanations for this disturbing trend, according to a major report from the Kaiser Family Foundation. For one thing, "the aging process itself seems to increase women's susceptibility to infection . . . possibly due to thinning of vaginal walls and abrasions resulting from insufficient lubrication." Sexual aids like Viagra may fuel the epidemic by prolonging some couples' sex life, but another significant reason is sociological. "Heterosexual women re-entering the dating field after twenty or thirty years" during which gender roles have changed are "not quite sure how to negotiate safe sex," says Kathy Nokes, chair of the New York Task Force on HIV. "This is a generation that didn't necessarily grow up thinking or talking about condoms," adds Monica Rodriguez, of the Sexuality Information and Education Council of the United States (SEICUS). "And most women over fifty aren't concerned about pregnancy." But they should be concerned about AIDS and other sexually transmitted diseases.

According to the venerable Kinsey Institute (see Chapter Seven), sex education is "sadly lacking" for the most rapidly growing segment of our society—the boomers. In many ways we are as misinformed as we fear our teenagers are. Most of us claim that we prefer to get information about sex from our physicians, but few of us do. We are woefully ignorant of the interrelationship between illness, treatment, the aging process, and social attitudes when it comes to sexual problems, and we are all too ready to put those problems into the what-I-can't-change category.

Moreover, physicians themselves don't know all we think

they do. In a stranger-than-fiction twist on the small-man paradigm, the next frontier in sexuality research is testosterone deficiency in postmenopausal women. The experience so far suggests that a testosterone supplement—available in Britain but not in the United States—can not only increase libido, but can stimulate energy, hair growth, and healthy nails. But when researchers tried to stimulate Viagra-like responses—a rush of blood to the genital area—in women, the results were inconclusive. The befuddled scientists realized that the physiology of our sexual response is unknown territory. Dr. Irwin Goldstein of Boston University School of Medicine admitted that there is a long way to go in the field. "It's odd to think about drugs when we don't even know how the vagina works yet," he says.

Lessons of the Hormone Replacement Therapy Controversy

And then there are the clinical surprises. The sudden cancellation of a major hormone study after adverse preliminary findings highlighted the danger of thinking we know what we need to know about a cure for what ails us. It is also an important example of the challenge to even the most conscientious consumer of medical information to keep up with scientific breakthroughs.

The study involved Prempro, a widely prescribed estrogen–progestin combination that subdued hot flashes, mood swings, vaginal dryness, and other symptoms of the decline in estrogen. Hormone replacement therapy was also reputed to perform other protective functions: lowering cholesterol, preventing osteoporosis, reducing risk of heart disease and Alzheimer's. Women with a predisposition to breast or uterine cancer were advised against the treatment, but many others went on HRT at menopause and never stopped. By the year 2000 more than seventeen million women—of the forty million who had reached menopause—were on HRT.

With news that the study was canceled because of early results showing an alarming increase in the risk of breast cancer, thousands of women quit the hormones cold turkey. Some found the withdrawal only minimally uncomfortable and were glad they did it; others were thrown by the loss of the hormone, and some of them went back on it; still others decided to stick with HRT because the sense of well-being they were experiencing was worth it to them. Dr. Lila Nachtigall, professor of obstetrics and gynecology at New York University Medical School and a pioneer in the field of hormone replacement therapy, admitted to a revised opinion about another supposed benefit, "We may have to modify or abandon our hope that HRT can provide heart disease protection . . ." she said. "But with women now living a third of their lives after the menopause, the health and quality of that life can't be ignored." And then she summed up the challenge for every woman and her doctor: "Individual women still have individual symptoms, histories, priorities, and risks . . . Each woman is entitled to an evaluation of her personal risks and benefits by a knowledgeable physician."

Since Dr. Nachtigall has been my gynecologist for over a decade and I had participated in one of the hormone studies she conducted, I made an appointment with her to analyze my particular situation. Beyond that, I always benefit from the subtext to any visit with her—that life is more than the sum of body parts. Over the years I have heard about her husband and children—her daughter is now in practice with her—her grandchildren (one of whom called in the middle of my visit to discuss the merits of a blue over a red bathing suit), her struggles with her weight, her struggles with the medical establishment over the best treatment for menopausal women. On one occasion we found ourselves together at an outdoor square dance, and she really got into the do-si-dos. Our wide-ranging conversation will, I hope, suggest the kind of personalized decision making a woman is entitled to expect to engage in with her doctor.

While she was examining me, we chatted with that awkward intimacy fostered by the dreaded stirrups between us. I brought her up to date on the state of my health. I also reported that I had taken a liver flush—a two-day cleansing of the intestines, gall bladder, and liver that involved, among other nauseating ministrations, swallowing enough epsom salts to kill a horse. Both my chiropractor/kinesiologist and a homeopathic healer had recommended it for its energizing results and for the possibility that it would reduce my cholesterol level (it didn't). Dr. Nachtigall was not impressed. She chewed me out for buying the hype. "One of the miracles of the body is that it cleanses itself perfectly; the only time you need to flush out your body is in preparation for a colonoscopy." She chewed me out for taking advice from anyone not trained in medicine. "If they were real healers," she huffed, "they would be doctors."

She is right about the danger of quacks out there, but I feel I am right, too, in believing that medical doctors aren't the only practitioners who know how to cure and strengthen the body. I have found a few people—chiropractors, nutritionists, homeopaths, spiritual healers—who have convinced me through what they say and how they work that they have a gift for tuning in to the rhythm of my body. I have felt it. I leave a good treatment feeling energized, and, yes, harmonized. We have worked on aches and pains—like the women-only thumb problem—that I wouldn't have taken to my internist. There have been times—particularly when I felt very sluggish—that they have been able to get my juices going with bodywork and nutritional supplements when a medical doctor was ready to write heavy-duty prescriptions. And in the case of my cracking and ridged nails, a condition I thought was in the what-I-can't-change department, vitamin E brought some improvement. So I'm not going to give up the hippie side of my well-being regimen, but I wouldn't take any chances either. Dr. Nachtigall knows that. She asks about the vitamins and herbs I am taking and notes them in my chart.

As always, my high cholesterol is where we begin. I have a family history of arterial disease and the high cholesterol makes me a statistically good candidate for a heart attack. I tell her that my internist has become very insistent about my taking a statin—a widely prescribed group of drugs that slow the production of cholesterol by the liver and enhance its ability to remove bad LDL cholesterol from the blood. I did try one brand a couple of years ago, but I didn't like the way it made me feel.

Dr. Nachtigall has always insisted that my good HDL cholesterol is so good that the ratio between it and the bad kind is excellent. Moreover, she believes that the estrogen I have been on for ten years helps keep the cholesterol in check. I brought along my most recent blood work, which put my LDL and HDL cholesterol levels at a ratio of 3:3. "That is incredibly normal," she said. "But the new recommendations reduce the highest acceptable LDL, even if the ratio is good. So we have to watch that. . . . You are not a clear cut case. Statins are very safe, but there is slight risk of liver and muscle problems."

I dressed and we moved to her office. The ensuing hour-long conversation ranged over all three areas of well-being, including what I can't change about my aging body. At one point she said, "The estrogen helped your hair." To which I responded mournfully, "Oh, you should have seen how thick it was when I was young!" She dismissed my protests with a brusque, "It would be a lot worse now without estrogen." Later when we talked about regular exercise, she asked about my weight. I confessed I had gained about ten pounds in the past year, after losing twenty-five. "It doesn't show," she said. I grabbed a handful of my "spare tire" in mute disgust. "Ah," she said, "as soon as you turn sixty that shows up. Nothing to do about it. But," she added emphatically, "you've got to take off those ten pounds. It's not healthy."

We zeroed in on what can be changed, and the wisdom of risking HRT in the context of my own medical/emotional/ lifestyle history.

"Let's see," she began, reviewing my chart. "In the middle of 1992, your estrogen levels had begun to drop, but you hadn't gone into menopause. You had anxiety and depression like crazy. You had headaches." Me? Depressed? Premenopausal? I was stunned. I remembered none of this. She wasn't surprised at my surprise. "One of the terrible things that happens with managed care is that you change doctors, so no one has records. Your doctor doesn't know, and you can't help him because you have forgotten you were depressed.

"You were still getting periods," she went on. "First you had depression, then the menopause. I see that a lot. At that time, before you went on anything, your cholesterol was very high! Six months later you were still depressed. I said this is the real thing—go on the study." At the time she was conducting a study for a new HRT that was well-received in Europe and South America and seeking FDA approval here. I soon was, according to her notes, "feeling much better." My cholesterol was down, and vaginal dryness had cleared up, too.

As part of the study, my bone density was checked periodically. "In 1993 you were 105 percent of normal," she says with something almost like personal pride. "That particular estrogen formula is so good for bones and you took it at the right time—the time of most bone loss. The next density was good, too. So I'm not worried about your bones, even if they go down from 105 percent to 100 percent."

The study concluded in 1995, but the approval process was slow, so I went off HRT. "Soon after," she reports in a *Dragnet* voice, "I got a call—you were depressed again. So I put you on Prozac, which you hated. So I said fine, let's go for another HRT."

We tried one brand, but "you did badly on it; it brought on hot flashes—which you have *never* had. Then we tried another—and you bled. Then we tried the one you have been on for the past three years." She seemed to be reviewing the bidding in her mind. "All estrogen is wonderful on cholesterol. The one you are on is not the perfect one, though. There is one that is better—it is the only oral estrogen that lowers triglycerides. The reason I want the oral form, not a patch, is the oral also increases HDL. So if this works without statins . . ."

"Is it any less dangerous than the others?" I asked.

"A little bit," she explained. "Because it is half the progestin. It is the same progestin—though a much lower dose—that is in birth control pills. There is a new study of norethindrone acetate which shows no increase in breast cancer after ten years."

"How's this on memory?"

"As good as you can do . . ."

I had one more question. "Is menopause any more idiosyncratic than other conditions?"

"First of all, you have to understand that menopause is a biological accident," she began. "We were only supposed to live to fifty. We outlived our biological destiny. Secondly, you have to understand that estrogen works in every organ of the body—you need it. Here and there it's a bad thing, mostly it's a good thing. It *is* idiosyncratic. There's a lot to look at. How is brain function? And memory function? How's your mood function and hair and skin and libido and vagina? And the picture changes. Some doctors say if you go on estrogen, you have to stay on it for the rest of your life. Why? We reevaluate it all the time. Is there a better drug? Are statins better than estrogen for you? Or do you need a little of each?"

For me, for now, HRT looks like the right way to go, in her opinion, for three reasons: "Your mood, your memory, and your vagina." It gave me confidence to know that she was basing her advice on adequate information about how my individual body works. It was up to me to take or leave her professional judgment, based on what I knew about her expertise. I decided that her recommendation was as good a body/mind/spirit package as I was likely to get.

The pieces of my well-being were coming together nicely that day. There was just one more thing: my nap. It is a secret indulgence. I lie down on the floor of my office and dose off in delicious privacy. Or I begin watching the six o'clock news and tune out for fifteen or twenty minutes. Needing a snooze in the afternoon is surely linked to the aging that I can't change but *taking it* is a definite step in the direction of what I can change. Most of all, the gift of not pushing myself—the way I did for all those years when I might have needed a nap but just never considered it—is the ultimate *wisdom* of listening to what my body is telling me.

CHAPTER TEN

Generations: Graduating from Our Child and Parent Voice to (at Last!) Our Own Adult Voice

Our strength and our anima stem in good part . . . from thinking about what it means to be a woman, here, now, in this culture, and in our imagined future. Our tribe is the tribe of woman.

—Natalie Angier, *Woman: An Intimate Geography*

My mother had me when she was twenty-five. I had my daughter when I was forty-four. I have colleagues and friends who are young enough to be my daughter—and old enough to be my daughter's mother. Many of my friends are grandmothers; we were born into the same demographic generation, but we have arrived at different generational roles. That puts me one generation after my mother, but in terms of age, two generations removed from my daughter. People occasionally do take me for her grandmother. Why, you may ask, do I even care about such arbitrary distinctions? For one thing the daughter–mother–grandmother sequence marks my progress along the traditional growth curve of a woman's life. At the same time the titles do the opposite. They codify the prescribed role expectations that have restricted a woman's growth. In my Second Adulthood I am struggling to understand both forces. I am trying to figure out where I am in the progression of my life and how someone my age can interact productively with a world that still categorizes women by the role they are considered old enough to play.

Psychologist James Hillman wisely observes that aging is about liberating *character* (what you do when you are alone) from *personality* (the traits you have developed to navigate society). Many of those traits have to do with the script we were given at each stage of life. The roles of mother, daughter, grandmother, sister account for much of the excess baggage—unresolved grievances, assumptions, deceit—we bring on this Second Adulthood journey. Replacing culturally defined roles with personal authenticity is the other half of the you-are-not-who-you-were-only-older equation.

Growing Up Together

Apart from the restrictive behavior imposed by tradition, generation does have meaning for us. We benefit from the reassurance that we have important elements of our personal history in common with others our age. A groundbreaking study—*Rocking the Ages*—by the Yankelovich Partners, a public research group, found that "members of a generation are linked through *the shared life experiences of their formative years*" more so than by personal experience or later stages of life. We are connected by the cultural language we learned and the shared memories of growing up in a particular time. There is a language barrier—though not an insurmountable one—between one generation and another.

I encountered this truth huddled in my sleeping bag on a barren island. Two days before the fabled cliff descent, our Outward Bound group was set down there to fend for itself—the infamous sine qua non of a wilderness challenge. On that cold uncomfortable night, I learned a little about survival and a lot about what sociologists call a *cohort*. From the time we dragged our duffel bags into a circle on the Maine shore three days earlier, I had been speculating idly about the age of one or another of my fellow campers. Most of them seemed to be in their thirties, a few in their forties and fifties, and one or two—including a former Navy Seal instructor—in their late sixties. But there was no correlation between the apparent age of anyone and their courage or stamina. Some were up to the hardest challenge, and others—like me—needed a boost over the climbing wall.

That night I was thrown headlong into a generation gap. After constructing makeshift lean-tos and feasting on fingers-full of peanut butter, we gathered around the one-match campfire and began to do what one does—tell tales and sing songs. The stories were fun to hear—I hadn't heard a good ghost story for years. Those few songs I recognized were fun to sing, but most were after my time. It was the laughter, though, that put me in my place. The thirty-year-old critical mass laughed about moments in TV shows I hadn't seen and about teenage fads that were unfamiliar to me, and they laughed themselves silly about condoms, of all things. Bemused, I thought of something poignant my immigrant father once admitted—although he learned to speak English comfortably, he never got the jokes. Humor comes with the territory; it is very hard to learn.

A few days later I would gratefully experience the gap from the other side—and from the specific perspective of my gender—in the almost wordless communion with those two other fifty-year-old women with whom I shared the exhilaration of saying no. The rest of the group had the shared experience of climbing back up the cliff; we had a shared epiphany in the language that only women of our age and place in time can understand.

Our Second Adulthood generation—spanning late forties, fifties, and sixties in age—is not an exact overlap with the baby boomer category (those born between 1946 and 1964), but it is illuminated by some of the characteristics the Yankelovich study singles out to distinguish that group from the generations before and after. Our collective past straddles the *matures* and the *boomers* and, especially in the workplace, comes into conflict with the *Xers*. The following are some distinguishing characteristics:

	MATURES	BOOMERS	XERS
Defining idea	duty	individuality	diversity
Celebrating	victory	youth	savvy
Work is . . .	an inevitable obligation	an exciting adventure	a difficult challenge
Leisure is . . .	a reward for hard work	the point of life	relief
Education is . . .	a dream	a birthright	a way to get ahead
Managing money	save	spend	hedge

Our "formative years" fall right between a culture of security and a culture of change. Our parents' generation never quite made peace with the insecurity of the out-with-the-old-in-with-the-new mood of the fifties. The generations that follow ours take progress for granted and consider change a way of life. We grew up on both sides of such major watersheds as jet travel, a television in every home, space flight, rock and roll, the computer, civil rights, and legal abortion. Between 1959 and 1961 (when all of us were young), the following defining events took place: the Barbie Doll, panty hose, the birth control pill, and Valium were introduced; JFK was elected president and the peace corps was started; the IBM Selectric type-writer and the *twist* dance craze hit; and Natalie Wood and Warren Beatty gave us the first on-screen French kiss in *Splendor in the Grass.* By 1968, the milestones were more disturbing: Martin Luther King and Robert Kennedy were assassinated, the My Lai massacre was uncovered, the Democratic convention and many college campuses erupted in violence. One bright spot of that year was the debut of *Mister Rogers' Neighborhood.*

We now work with people who can't imagine how a typewriter worked, who aren't sure which Kennedy was which, and if they know about student protests, they are tired of hearing about them. As the touchstones of our era lose their relevance to the culture at large and are replaced by others we don't always *get,* we will need to find new entry points into the world around us. We are no longer native speakers; for us, from now on, it is going to be the Culture as a Second Language.

Keeping the conversation going is more important to us than it was to any generation before, because we as a group intend to keep growing up with the generations around us. Instead of retreating to the porch to reminisce about the good old days, we have every intention of generating new experiences every day. Alongside the rest of the adult population.

We are crafting our generation's response to becoming old enough to be considered the adult world's grandmother. An alternative to the granny model will emerge, one that reflects the impulse many of us feel to make new connections with future generations. While we resist mightily being typecast as the indulgent, available-any-time babysitter in orthopedic shoes, we admit to marveling at the wonder of babies and to a growing consciousness of what we want them to know. This longer-range view inspires some of our most heartfelt answers to The

Question "What am I going to do with the rest of my life?" Isabella, the mother of an adopted and a biological child, makes a beautiful distinction between the two drives to connect with humankind. "My biological child connects me to my own genes, my dead parents," she says. "My adopted child connects me to humanity; there is a larger embrace."

When Margo decided to go into the Peace Corps with volunteers half her age, or Alexis realized she wanted to make her Second Adulthood an example for her children of "someone who embraces life," or Teri took on the mentoring of a recovering addict who was the age the child she never had would have been—they were embracing the generations around them. They are also creating roles for themselves that will stand as models for the younger women when they get to our stage.

In the course of recalibrating our most intimate relationships, we are examining our entanglements with generations before and after ours. We may be grandmothers, but we are not *only* grandmothers. We may be mothers, but the young women we work with are not our daughters. We may not be mothers, but we parent other people's children. We may be daughters, but we are also having to mother our long-lived mothers.

To manage all those relationships, we have learned to speak in three distinct voices: Each of us has a *child voice,* a *parent voice,* and—we hope—an *adult voice.* One of the first satisfactions of Second Adulthood is the sound of one's own adult voice speaking up forcefully and under circumstances in which we had until then been choking on a parent voice or a child voice. That is how we assert our rightful place in the world around us. Speaking across time and experience to other generations gives one's own voice resonance.

The Child Voice

As hard as it may be to see ourselves as society's grandmothers, it is that much harder to acknowledge that we are still our parents' daughters. Second adolescence and the Fuck You Fifties are also a second wave of rebellion. In the same way that Ruth and Karen encourage their Retirement or What Next groups to identify and silence the old voices of parental disapproval and control in order to hear their own voices, we may have to go through some of that adolescent pain again if we are to establish ourselves as free agents now. The most intense negotiation is between mothers and daughters, and it can take place even if our mothers are no longer alive. For some it can only happen *when* their mothers are no longer alive. Georgia, who never married or had children, called her mother "Mommy" until the day she died two years ago. She feels the "loss of childhood," the end of the beginning. "I was overwhelmed," she recalls, "with a sense of not aloneness, but on-your-ownness. I was nobody's little girl any more. It was the final push out of the nest." She remembers saying to herself as sternly as she could, "Girlfriend, if you weren't grown up before, you sure are now.

"There is a hole in my soul," Georgia admits mournfully. "I will always be her child. I liked being her child. But I understand that I am stepping up, that I am now *the* generation and I will never sit at the kids table again."

Psychologist Carol Gilligan was stunned to discover, in the days after her mother died, that "suddenly there was nothing between me and the horizon." A few weeks later, she was taking a dance class and glimpsed her characteristically disheveled hair in the wall-length mirror. "I realized that I was seeing my self with only two eyes, not the four eyes of me and my mother, she saying 'your hair,' and then, 'darling,' and then 'brush the hair away from your face,'" she writes.

Wrestling with parental expectations is to do combat with the assumptions from our first adulthood. Our mothers can't help but see—and love—that earlier persona, composed of the many imposed roles and attitudes that we now find problematic. Like Carol's mother, they all have an image of how we should look and behave and what we are good at. Jungian analyst James Hollis, who also recognizes the stages of first and second adulthood, points out a catch-22 of the readjustment process. In our Second Adulthood, he explains in *The Middle Passage: From Misery to Meaning in Midlife,* we are in a position to deal with our parents as equals—adults if you will—but at the same time we still need to "differentiate" ourselves from them in order to, as we so often put it, "grow up." As we struggle with our own identity, we associate our parents with one we have outgrown, "the false self . . . the provisional identity acquired during the first adulthood."

At the same time as we plumb the depths of our own being for sparks of authenticity, we look for whatever truth there may be in our perceptions of our mothers' lives. Every woman I interviewed measured her experience against her mother's. Some were positive; some were not. What I found was that many were revising their take on their mothers' experience as they revised their own outlook. Several talked about gaining new perspective on the choices their mothers made. Others felt they were better able to put those choices into a context that included both of them. Carol Gilligan came to the realization that "what I had thought of as just my difficulty in coming to grips with my relationship with my mother seemed part of a more general struggle on the part of women to undo a rewriting of history."

Stephany's mother had been an advertising copywriter before she married; she continued to work until she made more money than her husband. At that point, although she didn't have children yet, she quit her job and for the next thirty years kept house in the suburbs. But she remained "in her own way quite an independent person." She founded a League of Women Voters chapter in her community, she ran for mayor and lost by only six votes, and she read a lot. "She always read the *New York Times*," recalls Stephany; "she would say, 'I do that so I'll be interesting for your father.'"

"I have to tell you," she adds after a pause, "I think I felt sorry for my mother. I never wanted to live in a town like this"—the one Stephany now lives in—"and be stuck the way my mother was stuck." Despite the parallel, Stephany is devoting her Second Adulthood to doing what she now believes her mother was trying to do—move on. At one point, she recalls, her mother toyed with the idea of going back to work, but, she told her daughter, "'if I went back to work, I'd work with people your age . . .' Isn't that a sad thing?" She died at sixty-two, awaiting her husband's retirement. And looking back, Stephany muses, "I think that the last ten years or so were probably difficult for her in terms of 'now, what do I do?'" because she was mired in self-doubt. Stephany is determined to be proactive about that urgent question.

Alexis feels blessed to have a mother who was a model of warmth and accomplishment, who taught her daughters that taking care of one's self was as worthy a priority as self-sacrifice. A dynamo, her mother raised eleven children while employed full time, took flying lessons, and earned a degree in finance. "She was just a busy, busy, wonderful lady, and of course I credit everything I am, and hope to be, to my mom." But it is an "outrageous act" on her mother's part that Alexis cherishes now more than ever—the annual "fishing trip" her mother initiated. When she was in her late fifties and "up to her eyeballs with kids and work," and Alexis was a sophomore in college, her mother realized that they both "needed to get away." So she organized a lost weekend. "The two of us went up and got our manicures and our spas and had a wonderful time," Alexis remembers. "And then the following year we decided to involve my sisters." For the next thirty-six years Alexis, her four sisters, and their mother would take off once a year—"for a while people really thought we were fishing!" Now that their mother has died, the sisters keep up the practice and have included their sisters-in-law. Recently they took over a small bed and breakfast in upper Michigan. Needless to say, the restorative power is more than sybaritic. "It's a great time, a lot of talking and working things out, and catching up. . . . My brothers kind of stay in touch that way, too; you know—they go 'so what happened, what did you talk about?' "

Carole Hyatt's mom surprised her daughter with a totally out-of-character Second Adulthood reinvention. Widowed in her fifties, she was financially secure but felt lonely and irrelevant, Carole recalls. She had "never worked a day in her life," but she was determined to get a job. What, her daughter wondered, could she possibly get paid for doing? Simple, her mother explained. "The thing I like doing most is being a mother. I liked driving you and your brother around to lessons, and all that . . . so I'm going to be a nanny!" For six months she looked for a situation, with no success. One day, Carole, who makes her own living advising business women about career strategy, asked her, "How are you driving there?" "I'm taking my Cadillac" was the reply. "And what are you wearing?" "What I always wear." Carole suggested that she "dress for the part" and sure enough she landed a job soon after. "The only problem," Carole explains, "was that they also wanted her to clean up the kids' rooms. She said, 'I don't do cleaning.' So she brought her own housekeeper in, on a shared job—she had read about shared jobs" and they made it work for three years.

Carole's brother was "apoplectic" and tried to explain to his mother that she didn't "need the money." But, the proud nanny replied, "I'm not interested in the money; I'm interested in what the money stands for." With her first paycheck she bought lavish gifts for her grandchildren. When their parents protested, she exclaimed, "You don't get it. This is *my* money. And I can do anything I want with *my* money. I earned it." Unlike her brother, Carole does get it. "This unbelievable tale shows the enormous need—in her late fifties—to prove to herself that she had worth. And she did. I admired her greatly for that."

I have only recently begun to see that my own mother, whose feminine style I rejected so wholeheartedly, is, in fact, no shrinking violet. When I was growing up I found her beautiful and loving and supportive, but not in ways that I could imagine emulating. I saw her beauty and fashionable clothes as vanity, her devotion to the family as self-sacrifice, and her doting approval as too sweeping and indiscriminate. While I was aware that she took academic courses and played the piano and sculpted powerful figures in clay and that she loved to travel, I dismissed those interests as hobbies. My models were more assertive, more ambitious, more out there—men, in other words.

Now I see things differently. I see her courage and strength. In many ways she is a pioneering role model for Second Adulthood. Raised with two sisters and a brother in a small midwestern town by Polish refugee parents, she remembers her mother as fearful and hardworking. Her father, a window-washer, had a little more adventurous streak. The family struggled with day-to-day existence and she escaped into romantic dreams—of writing or acting, of a grand passion. My mother got herself to college—not just any college, but the iconoclastic University of Chicago of the late thirties—and then dropped out, moved to New York, and married a doctor, an old-world Hungarian who had no patience for romantics. They raised two children. My brother and I had established our own lives by the time our father died suddenly. My mother was fifty-one. Like many women of her generation, she was liberated by widowhood. What had been whispered background noise became her determined voice.

In the past thirty years, without any real encouragement or a support group of any kind, she has completed college, earned a master's degree in social work (working full time throughout) and at eighty-something got her Ph.D. All the while she has maintained her lifelong commitment to rescuing animals—venturing fearlessly into dark and dangerous basements in pursuit of a stray—and to political and civic activism, campaigning for candidates and threatening to run for office herself. Over those same years, she met and lost the love of her life and watched her son die of AIDS. And got through it. She did it all, and she did it all by herself. I admire her tremendously. I admire her guts, her stick-to-itiveness, her generosity, her laugh, and the way her response to a new idea is "That's really interesting."

What I can't stand is that she still babies me. "I am sixty years old!" I explode in adolescent-sounding exasperation, "old enough to . . . manage my health / drive in the rain / not call when I get there / give [blank] a piece of my mind." Not only too old to be babied, but not even a grown-up version of her baby. I am not who I was, only older, I try to explain, but it is hard to break through the accumulated assumptions we have about each other. I want her to know how much I admire her, but sometimes I think she is either not listening or not able to hear my overdue appreciation.

Recently, though, she has had to confront some of the inevitable problems of aging, and I am being forced to see the dynamic between us shifting: While for my own well-being I still need to get out from under her mothering, it is increasingly necessary—for *her* well-being—that I begin to mother her more. An unforeseen benefit to the long hours in doctors' waiting rooms is that we have more time to talk. During those desultory conversations, as she tells stories from her life and we discuss her plans for the future, I hear her voice differently. Maybe because I am less impatient—more mellow—about revisiting familiar family history. Maybe because I am on the same journey she is. In the same way as my second adolescence has put me in closer touch with my children's first adolescence, I think I am beginning to listen to my mother's reconsideration of her life less from the point of view of a rebellious daughter and more as a fellow traveler.

The Parent Voice

Because we are daughters and because we are women, the intensity of our relationship with our female children is carried to the umpteenth power. We adore our sons, and that relationship may become fraught with whatever ambivalent feelings we have about men, but they will always be *other*. Our own daughters are in many ways our doppelgangers. They are us, but with a mother who isn't making the same mistakes her mother made. They are us, but with a better chance at confidence, adventure, and success. They are also themselves—rejecting our attentions, cataloguing our mistakes, and keeping secret how much or how little they are like us.

By the time most women have reached their Second Adult-hood, they have reached some kind of equilibrium with their daughters. A modicum of space and authority has established itself. Most of the time. Like every other stage of parenting, though, just when you think you have got the house of cards up, the wind blows through. One mother is revisiting the an-guish of her daughter's adolescence as a runaway now that her daughter has moved back home with her two kids after her husband walked out. Another mother and daughter inherited a family business and are slamming doors in frustration with each other's way of doing things.

We are struggling to learn how, as a therapist who works with her clients on the three voices put it, "to parent an adult." One woman recognized that she and her daughter had made some important authority and space accommodations. "She's better able to set boundaries and I'm better able not to push," she said. "We are at that perfectly balanced point where neither of us is in charge of the other," said another mother. "While we are both interested in what each other's lives are like, there is a nice distance now—not exactly detachment, but mutuality—that increases rather than decreases our intimacy. I suppose," she adds thoughtfully, "when I get older that may change, but right now is the ideal balance between us."

A mother of two daughters and a son isn't quite there yet. Carolyn's daughters are eighteen and twenty-three. The younger one is "outgoing and funny, has a slew of nice friends, and ra-diates competence and good humor." The older one has "a darker aura. At age four, she told me that black was her favorite color. At fifteen she was kicked out of school. At twenty she was kicked out of college; she was experimenting with drugs and falling into a dysfunctional life—including at one point a disappearing act from which she emerged with a police record and a disastrous marriage." After two years of unspeakable anguish with the older daughter in and out of rehab and in and out of contact with her family, she has gotten back on track, and her mother is keeping her fingers crossed.

Carolyn still speaks in a parent voice. She finds both daughters "so much smarter, savvier, and more clued-in than I was at their ages that I glow with admiration and affection." But she admits, "I worry that their misfortune is somehow my fault, that bad luck seeks out the unlucky and the unwary, and is more likely to befall young women who have been encouraged—by their mother no less!—to experiment and to dare to be different."

Fran, whose thirty-five-year-old daughter is also in recovery from a long and heartbreaking struggle with addiction, has finally stopped worrying about what she did wrong. Her voice is more adult. "I can clearly see her strengths and weaknesses, but I no longer look for where they came from." When her daughter had a daughter, Fran found herself admiring the new mother. "I see her taking advantage of all being a mother has to offer. And she's a conscientious mother. She would never say, 'If you don't behave, I'm leaving and I'm not coming back!' as *I* did." Watching and remembering, Fran is forced to consider "what I might have been. There is hope—that Jennie will take advantage of what she has. And sadness—that I didn't."

With a daughter, says Fran, who also has a son, "you get those high estrogen moments that come from a shared history as women." Having a daughter and a granddaughter, she sees "the dance of life. When I change the baby's diaper I look at her bare little vulva and I see her in her mother's belly and her mother in my belly. And I wonder who will be in *her* belly. . . . And I miss my mother and wish that she were there."

Connecting to the Lives of Children
Not Your Own

"I couldn't imagine when I was young that I wouldn't have children, because I always liked them. But I never wanted to get married," admits Frida, a travel agent. "I was leading a really interesting life, traveling all over the world, meeting fascinating people." Nevertheless, children were an important factor in her life. "I think maybe if I didn't feel so close to my sister's kids I would have felt a great loss, but this is a wonderful redirection of the maternal instinct—without the responsibility."

Actually there is quite a bit of responsibility. Her sister was widowed when the children were young, so Frida paid for their schooling. "I was able to, and it was a thrill to be able to do it." The real thrill though has been the connection. "It was love at first sight with all of them. I probably didn't babysit that much, but I would visit them a lot. When they got old enough, three or four, they would come stay with me at my house for sleep-over dates, which was probably their first baby steps toward their own independence—leaving home, but . . ." As they got older, she shared her wanderlust with them. "I took them to historic places—to Washington and Williamsburg. I had always traveled on my own, because that was my job and my passion. But somehow taking the kids to places was really fun. I took my niece to Disney World when she was very little."

Frida is particularly close to that niece, who is now twenty-nine. "We looked exactly alike for years. We have a lot of the same interests—she's crazy about old movies, which is unusual in somebody that young. She loves Cole Porter, she loves the theatre, she's interested in politics, she's incredibly opinionated, even more so than I. I went to visit her often when she was in college, so I met most of her college friends. Now she's sort of self-contained about her feelings—but I'm still the person she has fun with."

"Aunt" Rosa's children aren't family members; they are children to whom she has made a serious commitment. She knows their favorite foods, their favorite teachers, and their friends as well as their parents do—and she knows a few things their parents don't. "Part of the deal," she says, "is that I will never violate a confidence." That commitment was sorely tested on one occasion. The teenage daughter of her closest friend, Sherri, came to Rosa. "'I'm pregnant,' she told me. 'And I don't want to have this child.' 'Have you told your parents?' I asked. And she said no, she couldn't. We talked about it a lot, but she wouldn't budge." So Rosa was left with a moral dilemma. "I had always told her she could come to me and trust me. But, I said to myself, holy moly, what do I do now? I called my sister; she said, 'Follow your heart.' So I helped her get that abortion."

For two years it was their secret, but then the teenager told a cousin, who in a spiteful moment told her parents. Rosa had taken a big risk not telling her friend Sherri at the time; she felt she was doing the right thing, but knew she might lose someone very important to her. When she found out, though, Sherri affirmed what Rosa calls the "circle of trust." "It was your decision, and I trust you to make that decision," Sherri told Rosa. "It wasn't your right to come to me. I'm just glad she had you to come to."

Finding an Adult Voice That Speaks to Younger Women

An important byproduct of the intergenerational intimacy with her niece, says Frida, is that it keeps her "connected to young people who work in this office, what their concerns are and how annoyed they can get at our generation. Because we certainly can be annoying."

We annoy each other most intensely when we assume a parent voice toward women who just happen to be young. "We are *not* your daughters," I heard over and over again from young professional and activist women who felt condescended to by the maternal assumption. "My first boss was a boomer woman who had no concept of where her power boundaries were," an outraged thirty-two-year-old told me. "She thought she could control me as a human being, and not just as a boss. Baby boomer women want to be your friend—it's not good enough to just do your job."

Realistically, it is unlikely that two women of different generations are going to be comfortable barhopping on a business trip or comparing notes on popular music. While younger women may have money hang-ups, they might never experience the bag lady syndrome or have difficulty saying no. We, in turn, will never experience their sense of entitlement, their sporting attitude toward sex, and their problem saying yes.

I am haunted by a line in Margaret Drabble's novel, *The Seven Sisters,* that captures the alienation that can develop between generations of women if we don't work at it. The main character, Candida Wilton, a fifty-five-year-old woman who has recently been divorced from her husband and estranged from her three daughters, moves to London to begin a new life. One of the first things she does is join a health club. But when she goes there she is crushed by the message she gets from the spry young attendants who look right through her. "To them I am an old woman," she sighs. "They do not know that I was once a child."

We need to listen to each other's stories as if we had never heard them before, no matter how much we believe we have. Because that is how we penetrate age barriers. It takes a degree of delicacy, and discomfort, to find the right tone in which to elicit those stories. A few years ago two young women I had worked with invited me to a dinner party for a couple of their friends and four or five "older women they admired." At first I was a little put off by the idea of being anyone's venerated elder. I anticipated an uncomfortable pressure to perform and be wise and, at the same time, I hoped to show them how hip and just-like-them I was. As it turned out, the evening was a lot of fun. The young women were full of energy, and it was touching to see how carefully they had planned the menu and the table setting. We reminisced about the "bad old days" of girdles and illegal abortions; they described modern-day sexism in action. We laughed—though not as much as if we had been in groups of our own age. We talked about our lives—though not as intimately as we would with contemporaries. And we went a little overboard praising each other's courageous acts of protest and daring. When it was over, I realized that I had been neither wise nor hip, but I had been engaged by the conversation. That felt good. We all felt good. But—I realize as I write this—my group hasn't reciprocated. We should. The tentative connection we made that night needs to be nurtured with the same devotion and delight that grandmas are expected to shower on their grandchildren.

Coming as we do from different times past, our understanding of what it means to be a woman will not always be compatible or even comprehensible to one another. But we mothers, daughters, aunts, and grandmas can forge a common vocabulary to share our perceptions. Our wisdom. We need to extend the courtesies of the new intimacy—acknowledgment of one another's authoritative (adult) voice and respect for the space between us. Because each of us needs to hear our own adult voice speaking the truth—to the present and to the future. What we make of the rest of our lives will depend in part on how each of us interconnects with the generations ahead and behind. An unanticipated legacy of our Second Adulthood may be an emotional framework for support and understanding among women that defies the artificial distinctions between generations and respects the real ones.

CHAPTER ELEVEN

Becoming a Critical Mass

The Personal Is Still Political

Such a critical mass of older women with a tradition of rebellion and independence and a way of making a living has not occurred before in history.

—Gerda Lerner, historian

Jyoti, the Jungian therapist who has studied native cultures around the world, had a dream about our generation. In it, she said, "we were donkeys and ponies, and we were a big dust storm going over the desert. Then, the dust settled and there was something new growing. That was what the wave of us had come to do. Until now, when we've gotten to a new stage, we've looked around and said, 'We don't like this; this is just crazy . . .' and we've changed it. Why should we use our elder years—our wise years—any differently?"

Saving the world is not what most of us have in mind for our Second Adulthood; even those like Joanne (see Chapter Six), who once did have that goal, have modified their ambitions somewhat. Yet the journey we are on—mapping our Second Adulthood—is taking us from a most intimate inquiry outward to the way we express ourselves in the world, the way we connect with other individuals and generations, and ultimately to the impact we can have on society.

Over and over, I met women who saw their Second Adulthood as a time for engagement with the world in ways that may or may not include the work they did before. Whether that means volunteering at a soup kitchen, or speaking out at a town council meeting, or mobilizing a "cousins club" to visit the family's country of origin; or whether it is a more time- and passion-consuming mission like bringing a referendum on an environmental issue, or raising funds for a needy arts insti- tution, or taking a paid position in a charitable organization; or something life-changing like starting a homeless shelter or bringing a lawsuit or running for office—the drive to connect is there. And the need is there.

We are part of a sea change that can lift a fleet of boats, not just our own. But we are only just beginning to become aware of the tidal wave we represent. Not only are we gaining strength both as individuals and as a group, but our influence is compounded by our attitude. "Women get more radical with age," Gloria Steinem frequently points out, because for one thing, we have had more years of experience coming up against false assumptions about what we are capable of, and for an- other, we have the daring that comes with the Fuck You Fifties to defy those barriers. Though we do not subscribe to a uni- form code of values or share similar aspirations, we each express our convictions and dreams loud and clear—in our votes, in our spending habits, and in the way we commit our time. Economists, politicians, corporate executives, sociologists, and medical researchers are waking up to the thundering herd of "ponies and donkeys" headed their way. And we should be too.

Indeed, most of the personal choices we make in answer to The Question will have an impact on the political and eco- nomic landscape. Whether we retire or postpone retirement or start our own business, travel or volunteer; whether we sell our homes or move in together; whether we abandon or embrace city life; and whether we move from one part of the country to another—all these individual choices will add up to a major impact on the demographics and economics of the country, dictating where roads are built, how airline routes are determined, the shape of congressional districts, and the way in which the nation's goods and services are distributed. We can let it happen or we can make it happen.

Throughout our first adulthood we experienced the validity of the phrase "the personal is political"; what made one woman feel stifled, oppressed, or just uncomfortable, often to her own shame, would turn out to be part of a larger pattern that needed to be changed. And then, no longer isolated and guilt-ridden individuals but an activist lobby of dissatisfied citizens, we set about to change it. Just remember how the inability of thousands of young athletes to get themselves taken seriously created the groundswell that opened up Little League competition to girls and produced Title IX legislation. The potential for that kind of cultural shift exists today. We can become an agent for change, and—thanks to the Second Adulthood housecleaning we have been doing in our lives— we can focus our energies on any cause we choose. Thirty-seven million doses of "postmenopausal zest" make quite a potent brew.

A sixty-four-year-old college dean I know worries about the impact a group as resourceful and demanding as ours could have if it is focused exclusively on its own interests. As she contemplates her own retirement, she warns that "if we are not careful, we will suck all the oxygen out of the system." That our success might siphon resources away from other equally needy but less influential groups is a real concern. But we are also in a position to put some oxygen *back* into the system. We have the voting power, economic clout, the leadership skills, and the organizing experience to reshuffle the priorities of our society—and not just for ourselves.

Voting Power

Every politician has an eye on us. The so-called gender gap—the divergence of women's votes from men's—was first observed just as some of the youngest of us were voting for the first time. In 1971, a poll by the Louis Harris Organization—commissioned by Virginia Slims cigarettes to confirm its "you've come a long way, baby" slogan—showed a growing unrest and assertiveness among women voters. Harris found that "there are signs that women are now playing for keeps in politics, more than any time in the past, and that this activism will accelerate." The numbers confirmed a "growing confidence, determination and bitterness that combine to make a potential explosion of woman-power in American politics." Over the next thirty years—our first adulthood—the trend has solidified, and the gap has been shown to increase with age.

That wasn't all Harris observed. In the same way our methods of solving problems and doing business are recognized as distinctively collaborative and holistic, so is our political vision. Women are "more inclined . . . to vote and to become active not only for their own self-interest, but for the interest of society, the world, and most of all, out of compassion for humanity," he reported. Since then, the pattern has been documented over and over again. Polls show that the issues women consider priorities—abortion, the environment, gun control, social programs—are lesser concerns for men. In general, we envision a government that takes responsibility for providing basic services to the community. Ethel Klein, who runs a strategic research firm that advises candidates, sees the issues gap in terms of the female experience. "Historically, men feel they've done it on their own—or should have—while women know they didn't, that you need community to succeed."

Over the same time women have been entering politics—moving from the PTA to the statehouse to Congress—in growing numbers. As activist and Congresswoman Bella Abzug proclaimed during her 1970 campaign, "This woman's place is in the house—the House of Representatives." Here too, Klein sees a distinctly female motivation in women candidates. "Women," she finds, "enter politics in order to make change and solve problems." More women are in office today than ever before. Are we holding them to those better instincts? As a matter of fact, are we holding ourselves accountable for our own votes? (The momentum is already there. In 2000, when barely half the electorate turned out, two-thirds of women in our age group did.)

As women become an increasing majority of voters, and Second Adulthood women become an increasing proportion of that group, the political process will begin to reflect the potential for change we represent. In response to the economic and military crises that have heated up since the turn of the new century, many of the women I talked to were toying with the idea of becoming more active in politics. Most saw their participation in terms of rounding up votes for a candidate in the existing system, but few are fully aware of how our voting power could be mobilized on behalf of a gender-gap agenda that could bring forward new leaders.

Economic Clout

We are now in the unprecedented position of being able to put some money where our big-mouth opinions are. The more

equitable our earning power becomes and the more knowledgeable we become about financial management, the more
money we have to spend and invest. (Forty-eight percent of
U.S. shareholders are women and they own 53 percent of the
stock.) We are becoming a source of capital and enterprise,
and we are becoming a major consumer bloc, too. We can
make a big difference by simply putting our dollars behind
causes or people that seem to have the right idea, or we can
make investments and purchases with those concerns in mind.

Our buying power is particularly potent. You wouldn't know
it to look at the ads, in which we are invisible, but we spend
one-third more on toiletries ($8 billion) than women eighteen
to thirty-four and, according to *Women's Wear Daily*, the apparel industry bible, "industry representatives confirmed that
despite being ignored by many marketers, graying boomers are
the most powerful force in the apparel industry." Harvard Business School professor Shoshana Zuboff, who runs a program
called Odyssey: School for the Second Half of Life, has come
to the conclusion in her book written with James Maxmin,
The Support Economy, that the challenges of our tumultuous
lives so far puts us "in the vanguard of the new society of individuals, even as it amplified [our] role in consumption." That
suggests, she goes on, "that the commercialization of women's
dreams will be an important factor in the next economic revolution . . ." What those dreams are and how they are com-
mercialized are questions we need to answer before economic
forces do it for us.

We have yet to harness the consumer power of our Second
Adulthood, but it offers a wide range of opportunities for
activism—the very successful first consumer boycott was organized in 1973 by housewives over meat prices—and for entre-
preneurship with a message. Anita Roddick, now sixty-one, who

built the Body Shop into a $1.37 billion a year operation, has demonstrated how influential a businesswoman can be when she decides to connect profits with politics—and when like-minded consumers back her up with their purchasing power. Roddick's approach to business is that it is "primarily about human relationships." The company focuses on taking "stakeholders" into the decision-making process and in turn urging customers that "it is the responsibility of every individual to actively support those who have human rights denied to them." It also lobbies for a wide range of causes, and Roddick hopes the Body Shop will serve as a model and "lead the way for businesses to use their voice for social and environmental change."

Leadership Skills

While it is possible to underestimate our political or economic clout, our emergence in positions of authority has not gone unnoticed. More than ever, women are making decisions at the highest levels. And the skills they bring to the job are being recognized as especially effective in meeting the challenges of the technological and global marketplace: Sharing of information horizontally, problem-solving that calls upon the expertise of those engaged in the enterprise, and the ability to improvise tactics as the circumstances arise. Interdependence, our most comfortable working model, is a primary requirement for participating in what Peter Drucker, the father of modern management, calls the new *knowledge economy* where skilled workers "are not amenable to" being ranked hierarchically but must be "linked." As Helen Fisher points out in *The First Sex,* "the expansion of telecommunications . . . has undermined the ability of a few people at the top to broker or withhold vital information and connections."

Like Roddick, Meg Whitman, forty-seven, the widely respected CEO of the successful online auction service eBay, has made interactivity her management style. A staff meeting sounds more like a community speak-out than a council of generals. "She insists that other executives voice their opinions on troublesome issues before she expresses her own," reports the *New York Times* in a business profile. "By all accounts she listens carefully but does not hesitate to overrule her colleagues." Her business philosophy is that success lies in focusing on and engaging the company's constituency. eBay solicits feedback from users, and Whitman has instituted regular "voice of the customer" sessions where a cross section of buyers and sellers are brought to headquarters for two days of talks with executives. That is the quintessential grassroots model. It gets the people affected by an institution invested in the process, and invests the process with their energy and ideas. We have used that model very effectively in the past. Only then we were on the outside looking in.

Organizing for Change

So much of our experience with the world at large has been shaped by being outsiders that we have trouble accepting and taking advantage of the fact that many of us are now power brokers and decision makers in realms that once seemed off-limits. And perhaps because so many of us are more comfortable on the inside these days, we have lost track of the continuing need to work on social problems from the outside in as we did so effectively in our first adulthood.

The women's health movement, which took shape in the early seventies, shows how the personal became political, and then powerful. Back when concern about how the medical establishment treated women began to coalesce around drugs like DES (diethylstilbestrol) and the Pill, most women only saw male doctors, scientific studies were conducted on male subjects—the small man principle (see Chapter Nine)—and conditions peculiar to women were hardly studied at all. Drug manufacturers spoke only to government agencies (in confidential reports and negotiations) and to doctors, who prescribed medications but never explained why, or what the risks were. Our expertise, even about our own bodies, was disregarded along with our wishes. "You have to remember," recalls Barbara Seaman whose groundbreaking *The Doctor's Case Against the Pill* was published in 1969 and helped trigger the women's health movement, "in those days doctors wouldn't let women have natural childbirth. They hit you on the head with anesthesia, and you weren't awakened until the hairdresser showed up."

We owe any mastery we have achieved over our own health management to the efforts of Seaman and her sisters-in-arms. The strategy was established early on: Energize a grassroots constituency that lacked a voice; create coalitions from smaller autonomous groups (mobilized around particular conditions, or the needs of a particular demographic group, or local issues); share strategies, contacts, and information through informal but efficient networks; and form alliances with sympathetic sources on the inside of government, industry, and the profession. And there was one more thing. "We made it a rule to take no money from those who might expect their pound of flesh in return," Seaman remembers. "Otherwise grassroots turns into Astroturf."

Although our medical problems are not yet getting the attention they deserve, women's health interests are now on the public agenda. They are there, because women whose medical needs have been neglected are demanding attention, because women's health has become a field with a body of information that professionals have to be aware of, and because women consumers have become active participants in their own care. Today there remain urgent societal problems in need of a movement. One of them strikes particularly close to home.

The Caregiving Crisis

At the same time as we are generating an explosion of energy that is changing our world, we are leaving an implosion of equal force in our wake. In that sense my friend is right to worry; we *are* sucking an important source of oxygen out of the system—the caregiving element. We are in the midst of what political scientist Mona Harrington calls a *social crisis* in which "the old formulas" of caregiving are "bankrupt." It is not our fault, but it is a direct result of choices we made.

Traditional assumptions about women's responsibility for taking care of everyone else—including in the community, where she is expected to donate time to the school, the library, the church—have led to some of the most painful moments in our first adulthood. Guilt, anger, and regret are intertwined with the trade-offs we made that gave us confidence and satisfaction. Now as we ease ourselves out of "the emotional management business" the caregiving system that relied on the unpaid or low-paid work of women is falling apart.

Existing institutions—schools, emergency rooms, shelters, even prisons, and families themselves—were not designed or funded to handle the needs of increasing numbers of citizens and are being crushed under the burden. "The fact is," Harrington writes in *Care and Equality*, "the old formulas cannot yield both care and equality. They are bankrupt. And they are generating a social crisis that cannot be addressed realistically until we can remove the blinders of traditional thinking and take in the whole of what is happening."

Is there anyone better positioned to remove the blinders of traditional thinking about caregiving than us? Even when women began to break out of the domestic framework, they—we—never broke free of that traditional thinking. We tried to do it all, to hold up both halves of the universe. The struggle to balance the two has defined our generation. And that hasn't changed, because the system hasn't changed. Every day women are missing work—and one third of them are losing pay—to care for a sick child. Twenty percent of them don't have health insurance. We have negotiated with men to share the load, but even two people are hard pressed to hold a job and care for children and—as 22.4 million families, nearly one in four, do—care for older family members or friends as well. It is even harder to stand up and say, "we can't and we shouldn't have to do this all by ourselves anymore."

"You have *got* to be kidding!" I can hear both my first and my Second Adulthood selves protest. "I spent the first half of my adult life feeling responsible for everyone but myself. I've finally discovered how to let go of the excesses of that experience. I'm only just beginning to care for myself. And now I'm supposed to get involved in creating a better system for caregiving with a capital C because I know so much about it!" I admit there is a certain irony to the suggestion that a mission of our collective Second Adulthood should be to pick up the pieces of the system that we just broke out of. But looked at another way, the same ethic of interdependence that made care for others such a priority, also gives us a model for a wider social net of community support. Add to that what we are learning about autonomy and interconnectedness—and about guilt reduction—and you have a starting point for a social policy that takes some of the caretaking responsibilities out of the individual homes and puts them into a societal framework that involves the whole community.

Our generation is the nation's "only increasing natural resource," contends Marc Freedman who runs a nonprofit group called Civic Ventures in San Francisco that addresses social policy issues. Because we have the energy, the time, and the know-how, we "are poised to become the new trustees of civic life in America," says Freedman. Our response to that challenge lies in the commitments—practical and spiritual—each of us makes to the rest of her life. When we ask ourselves, *What Matters?*, one response has to be "my community"—however each of us defines it. When we ask *What Works?*, we know the answer: A combination of participation, passion, and power. And when we ask *What's Next?*, we want to answer, "We're working on a better way!"

CHAPTER TWELVE

Riding the Spiral

At this time in our history, we should take nothing personally.
Least of all ourselves.
Try to do
whatever you do as an act of celebration.
WE ARE THE ONES WE'VE BEEN WAITING FOR.

—Hopi Nation, "Wisdom of the Elders"

When I began this book I thought of it as a journey, my journey to Second Adulthood. Now that I've gotten to the end of the book I see there is no end to the journey. Until, of course, the ultimate The End. But the book and I have come to a parting of the ways, and I hate to let it go. I don't want to give up the sense of purpose and focus that the years of talking and thinking and writing about the experience of Second Adulthood has given to my life. And I am apprehensive about going back to actually experiencing it. Back where I don't know what's coming next. Back where relationships are messy and consequences are unpredictable. Back where I can't rewrite what doesn't work. Where I can't call an expert to make sense of what is going on. Back where the best one can hope for is two steps forward and only one step back. Back where The Question, in its many forms, lurks. But one thing I do know. I know that as I write the end of this book I am not who I was at the beginning, only older. As a result, this transition to whatever is next for me feels more organic than earlier ones.

While the prospect of change is still disconcerting, it is no longer the destabilizing danger I fought so hard against. The journey so far has made me much more comfortable with change as a lost-and-found process.

I have found courage among the women I talked to who were as brave and articulate and honest as I could ever hope to be. I have lost my nerve on occasion, sometimes about silly things, like telling my age—though I turned from almost sixty-one to almost sixty-two, I still say I'm just sixty. I have experienced incredible highs of creativity when I amazed myself with the way my ideas were fitting together. And lows, when I felt old and fat and stupid. But even in those depths, I came to trust the process—if I let things percolate, they will most likely fall into place. I have lost whole days of work in anguish over a family problem, as I have all my working life, but there were other days when I was able to say, "It's not my problem. I can't fix it," and move on. I learned something about how the brain works and how anthropologists think. And then—with some prodding—I forced myself to say what *I* think.

I have let my memberships lapse in the professional organizations of my first adulthood life. I finally believe that I have found a new calling. Because I've spent so much time alone, I've definitely lost some social graces. I'm more clumsy than ever at small talk, but I have delivered some feisty comebacks and become more adept at drawing people out. I have kept my workout schedule, but I have definitely lost all pretense to chic. I am totally embedded in sweatpants and T-shirts and my feet have grown hooves at the heels from wearing nothing but clogs. I'm going to try to get some style back in the next phase.

As I say "the next phase," I realize that I now see my life in more episodic terms than before. I even count on the coming-around-again rhythm my Second Adulthood has taken on. When I started out, like most of us, I was looking for blueprints and strategies that would show me what to do with the rest of my life. What I found is energy and confidence and community but more questions than answers. Most important, though, all the revisiting and redefining and recalibrating has prepared me to accept that the journey itself is a recycling process.

In her book about reinvented lives and "multiple fresh starts," Mary Catherine Bateson reminds us "that there is always something in the past to work with." Each of the women she wrote about found that "she has enough experience of new beginnings to be skilled in recycling what she has learned in new contexts . . . We have learned from interruptions and improvised from the materials that came to hand, reshaping and reinterpreting."

We're *re*shaping and *re*interpreting our way through the Fertile Void and toward a *re*discovery of our passion and our voice and our mastery. We're *re*vitalizing our bodies. We're *re*configuring a new kind of intimacy with those close to us and *re*constituting our connectedness to the human family. Every day we are in the process of *re*inventing ourselves.

Process, we are beginning to understand, *is* progress. It is messy and rambling, even retrograde, at times, but Second Adulthood pulses with life. The best evocation of the force building within us that I have found is in Quincy Jones's description of the music—music that is both improvisational and purposeful—that moves him. "Jazz," he writes in his autobiography, "conditioned me not to be a rigid thinker, to have my mind constantly open. You need to improvise on life. . . . Jazz . . . shapes how you deal with people, how you love people. It's about freedom, imagination, and being able to shift on a dime. It's a totally nonrigid, democratic perspective on the world."

Every one of the women I met feels jazzier now than when she first fell into the Fertile Void. Take Margo, who was so happily ensconced in her Peace Corps village in the Ivory Coast. Since I introduced her at the start of this book, the government there was overthrown and foreign nationals evacuated. She had to "shift on a dime." Now back in the United States and trying to find a new answer to The Question, she is still experiencing almost "no static on the line." The faith in the process that came with the big change she made in her life seems to be here to stay. "I have given away my entire household and most of my clothes," she says of her hurried departure. "I'm storing the rest. Either I'll forget about it or come back when things calm down."

Or Eliza, a country/new age singer who is fifty-three. "Right now I'm so clear about what I'm doing. I feel like I'm flying," she says. But the lead-up to her fiftieth birthday set off a grieving process. "I had to let go of what I call *false powers*— the power to manipulate men; the power of youth. I realized that one day you push on that gas pedal and nothing happens." Nowadays, she says, her priority is reclaiming her true power. "I don't want to live with a man again until I can take care of myself, financially, emotionally, and nurturingly." She understands that there is no direct route to that kind of goal. "My worst days are when I feel I'm stuck in the same old pattern that I'm doomed to repeat. That I'll just dry up." But recognizing the pattern—"I can see it coming now," she says—is in itself a breakthrough. With each encounter, the pattern is weaker and Eliza is stronger.

Like Eliza, each of us is making circles around our experience, yet with each cycle we attain a little more perspective and a little more lift. The ingredients shift in importance, the risks change in character, the passions surge and ebb, and we swoop and soar among the currents. Joanne, who found her voice when she reconnected to her body, describes the joy of discovery in motion. "As I danced, I learned to roll my hips, awkwardly at first, and then with relish if not grace. My arms reached out, and my legs grew strong. I found circles in my body that I had never known were there."

I realize how far improvising—to use Quincy Jones's word— has taken women like Margo and Eliza and Joanne and me, when I encounter someone just starting out. Not long ago television journalist Jane Pauley announced to her stunned employers and admirers that after twenty-seven years at NBC, she was leaving the job. Why? Because, she said, at fifty-two she was ready to "reshape" her life. Her twins had just gone off to college and a six-month sabbatical after her fiftieth birthday had been refreshing. I could almost hear her engines revving up as she described how she came to the decision. "Women think a lot about cycles, biological and personal," she said. "This year another cycle came around; my contract was up. It seemed like an opportunity to take a life audit." I had a flashback to the image of myself rappelling down that cliff five years ago and landing in the Fertile Void when Pauley admitted that she had no idea "what's next, or even, what do I really want to do." Welcome to Second Adulthood, girlfriend. You are in for a great ride!

What was once unknown territory is becoming familiar to more and more women. And, as we have learned so dramatically in our first adulthood, when we share our experience, we clear the underbrush along the path for each other.

I hope this book can function as a circle of trust for the reader. It did for me. The women I interviewed were generous with their stories, and I have tried to share the wisdom of what they said. We have learned that nuggets of truth and humor are what get us through the night. Each of us listens to another woman's life in terms of our own, and each takes away her own inspiration. We underline different sentences of the same paragraph.

In the course of the many conversations I had, an occasional phrase or insight spoke directly to me, tidbits that I wanted to post on the refrigerator door of my mind. They are like postcards from the journey so far.

The reminder on Joanie's handicraft mirror—"no need to sparkle"—comes upon me regularly and makes me smile with gratitude. The notion of going out of the emotional management business has been a beacon of clarity on occasions when I was sinking into the morass of trying to ensure that everyone I love is happy. And Elizabeth's no-nonsense response to waking up in the middle of the night and berating herself with woulda-coulda-shoulda regrets is a bracing and reliable piece of advice. She simply tells herself sternly to "shut up" and goes back to sleep.

As the mother of an adopted child and a biological child, I am inspired by Isabella's observation that her biological child connects her to her family tree, and her adopted child connects her to the human family. I found a profound affirmation of the friendships I cherish in Vivi's description of her bedside visits to a dying friend: "I know it's a great burden on someone who's not well to interact with a visitor, so I told her, 'You don't have to talk when I come; we've talked our whole lives. I'll just be with you.'" And there is an equally profound sense of wonder at womanhood in Fran's musing as she contemplated her new granddaughter's vulva and tried to imagine the future. I also love her use of that slightly risqué word—*vulva;* it celebrates the outspoken daring of the Fuck You Fifties that I find so liberating.

Being a work in progress means living with the two-steps-forward and one-step-back nature of the creative process, and finding stability in the rhythmic and reliable ebb and flow itself. "Intermittency" is what Anne Morrow Lindbergh called it in *Gift from the Sea,* written fifty years ago. Despite the instability of life's course that she concedes is almost "impossible" to accept, she found magic in the equipoise between the contradictory currents, "where the breathlessly still ebb-tides reveal another life below the level which mortals usually reach. In this crystalline moment of suspense, one has a sudden revelation of the secret kingdom at the bottom of the sea." And security in the dynamic of the moment, "neither in looking back to what it was in nostalgia, nor forward to what it might be in dread or anticipation, but living in the present . . . and accepting it as it is now."

Stephany had a similar insight about a definition of middle age that she found intriguing—"when a person begins to think of time in terms of how long until they die, rather than how long since they were born." In her experience, the emphasis is somewhat different. "I don't sit around and think when am I going to die, but I often think: it's like OK. This is where I am."

That aspect of the dynamic—the stasis within motion—is the final piece of the puzzle for me. It explains the sense of peace—mellowness—we experience in the midst of so much flux. How is it that we keep recreating familiar patterns and at the same time feel we are breaking out of old constraints? How is it that we long to set goals yet feel more alive when we are reconsidering them? How is it that the more we are in flux the more grounded we feel? That the further we get from who we were, the closer we get to who we are? Early on, the sense of going around in circles is a frustrating symptom of the Fertile Void, but those circles look very different in later stages of the journey. Embracing. We start to see them as one element of a spiral—a circle plus change—that we are riding. And in the middle, held aloft in the whirlwind, is the person each of us truly is.

As we move from day to day, we realize we can ride the spiral but we cannot harness it. We can put ourselves in charge of some of that process; nature is in charge of the rest. Yet the momentum is clear: Instead of going around in smaller and smaller circles as tradition dictates a woman my age should do, and instead of retreading old dreams and assumptions as some of the cheerleaders for this age urge us to do, I now see myself riding upward and outward. As I look down, I see—and appreciate—the reassuring familiarity of my life so far. At the same time, each loop of my trajectory takes me somewhere I haven't been, to something I can only know when I get there.

Bibliography

Almeida, David M., "Stress Is Less When You're Older." *AARP Bulletin Online.* October 2002.

Angier, Natalie. "Weighing the Grandma Factor; In Some Societies, It's a Matter of Life and Death." *New York Times.* November 5, 2002, p. F1.

———. *Woman: An Intimate Geography.* New York: Anchor Books, 2000.

Appelbaum, Eileen and Rosemary Batt. *The New American Workplace: Transforming Work Systems in the United States.* Ithaca, NY: ILR Press, 1994.

Applewhite, Ashton. *Cutting Loose: Why Women Who End Their Marriages Do So Well.* New York: HarperPerennial, 1998.

Apter, Terri. *Secret Paths: Women in the New Midlife.* New York: W. W. Norton, 1995.

——— and Ruthellen Josselson. *Best Friends: The Pleasures and Perils of Girls' and Women's Friendships.* New York: Three Rivers Press, 1998.

Bach, David. *Smart Women Finish Rich: 9 Steps to Achieving Financial Security and Funding Your Dreams.* 2nd ed. New York: Broadway Books, 2002.

Bateson, Mary Catherine. *Composing a Life.* New York: A Plume Book, 1990.

Bauer-Maglin, Nan and Alice Radosh, eds. *Women Confronting Retirement: A Nontraditional Guide.* Piscataway, NJ: Rutgers University Press, 2003.

Benes, Francine M., Mary Turtle, Yusuf Khan, and Peter Farol. "Myelination of a Key Relay Zone in the Hippocampal Formation Occurs in the Human Brain During Childhood, Adolescence, and Adulthood." *Archives of General Psychiatry,* Vol. 51. June 1994, pp. 477–84.

Blum, Deborah. *Sex on the Brain: The Biological Differences Between Men and Women.* New York: Penguin Books, 1997.

Bolen, Jean Shinoda. *Crones Don't Whine.* York Beach, ME: Conari Press, 2003.

———. *Close to the Bone: Life-Threatening Illness and the Search for Meaning.* New York: Touchstone, 1996.

Boston Women's Health Book Collective, The. *Our Bodies, Ourselves for the New Century.* The Boston Women's Health Book Collective. New York: Simon & Schuster, 1998 [new edition projected for 2005].

Butler, Robert N. and Myrna I. Lewis. *The New Love and Sex After 60.* Revised ed. New York: Ballantine Books, 2002.

"By the Numbers: A *Newsweek* Poll on Aging." *Newsweek* Special Issue. Fall/ Winter 2003, pp. 9–10.

Canyon Ranch, staff of, with Len Sherman. *The Canyon Ranch Guide to Living Younger Longer.* New York: Simon & Schuster Source, 2001.

Carpenter, Candice. *Chapters: Create a Life of Exhilaration and Accomplishment in the Face of Change.* New York: McGraw-Hill, 2002.

Clinton, Hillary Rodham. *Living History.* New York: Simon & Schuster, 2003.

Covey, Stephen R. *Seven Habits Of Highly Effective People: Restoring the Character Ethic.* New York: Firestone, 1989.

Damasio, Antonio. *The Feeling of What Happens: Body and Emotions in the Making of Consciousness.* New York: Harcourt, 1999.

De Mille, Agnes. *Martha: The Life and Work of Martha Graham.* New York: Random House, 1991.

Diesenhouse, Susan. "At Home with: Joan and Robert B. Parker; A House Divided, Lovingly." *New York Times.* August 23, 2001, p. F1.

Drabble, Margaret. *The Seven Sisters.* New York: Harcourt, 2002.

Dreifus, Claudia. "Sense & Sensuality." *AARP Modern Maturity.* November/ December 2002, pp. 40–44.

Drucker, Peter F. *The Essential Drucker.* New York: HarperBusiness, 2001.

Dychtwald, Ken. *Age Power: How the 21st Century Will Be Ruled by the New Old.* New York: Jeremy P. Tarcher, 2000.

Erikson, Erik H. *Identity and the Life Cycle.* New York: International University Press Inc., 1959.

Erikson, Erik H. and Joan M. Erikson. *The Life Cycle Completed: Extended Version.* New York: W. W. Norton, 1998.

Fisher, Helen. *The First Sex: The Natural Talents of Women and How They Are Changing the World.* New York: Ballantine Books, 1999.

Freedman, Marc. *Prime Time: How Baby Boomers Will Revolutionize Retirement and Transform America.* New York: Public Affairs, 2000.

Friedan, Betty. *The Fountain of Age.* New York: Simon & Schuster, 1993.

———. *The Feminine Mystique.* New York: W. W. Norton, 1997 [1963].

Gersick, Connie and K. E. Kram. "High-Achieving Women at Mid-Life: An Exploratory Study." *Journal of Management Inquiry,* Spring, 2002, pp. 104–27.

Gilligan, Carol. *The Birth of Pleasure.* New York: Knopf, 2002.

———. *In a Different Voice: Psychological Theory and Women's Development.* Cambridge, MA: Harvard University Press, 1993.

Gleick, James. *Faster: The Acceleration of Just About Everything.* New York: Pantheon Books, 1999.

Goode, Erica. "A Conversation with Daniel Kahneman; On Profit, Loss and the Mysteries of the Mind." *New York Times.* November 5, 2002, p. F1.

Goodman, Ellen and Patricia O'Brien. *I Know Just What You Mean: The Power of Friendship in Women's Lives.* New York: Simon & Schuster, 2000.

Guiliano, Mireille. "The Boss; No Hiccups in Risk Taking." *New York Times.* November 8, 2000, p. C8.

Gutmann, David. *Reclaimed Powers: Men and Women in Later Life.* 2nd ed. Evanston, IL: Northwestern University Press, 1994.

Hanauer, Cathi, ed. *The Bitch in the House: 26 Women Tell the Truth About Sex, Solitude, Work, Motherhood, and Marriage.* New York: William Morrow, 2002.

Hansell, Saul. "Meg Whitman and eBay, Net Survivors." *New York Times.* May 5, 2002. section 3, p.1.

Harrington, Mona. *Care and Equality: Inventing a New Family Politics.* New York: Knopf, 1999.

Heilbrun, Carolyn G. *The Last Gift of Time: Life Beyond Sixty.* New York: Ballantine Books, 1997.

———. *Writing a Woman's Life.* New York: Ballantine Books, 1988.

Hillman, James. *The Force of Character and the Lasting Life.* New York: Random House, 1999.

Hochschild, Arlie Russell. *The Time Bind: When Work Becomes Home & Home Becomes Work.* New York: Metropolitan Books, 1997.

Hollander, Linda. *Bags to Riches: 7 Success Secrets for Women in Business.* Berkeley, CA: Celestial Arts, 2003.

Hollis, James. *The Middle Passage: From Misery to Meaning in Midlife.* Toronto: Inner City Books, 1993.

Jolly, Alison. *Lucy's Legacy: Sex and Intelligence in Human Evolution.* Cambridge, MA: Harvard University Press, 1999.

Jones, Quincy. *Q: The Autobiography of Quincy Jones.* New York: Doubleday, 2001.

Jong, Erica. *Fear of Flying.* Austin, TX: Holt, Rinehart and Winston, 1973.

Legato, Marianne J. *Eve's Rib: The New Science of Gender-Specific Medicine and How It Can Save Your Life.* New York: Harmony Books, 2002.

Lerner, Harriet. *The Dance of Anger: A Woman's Guide to Changing the Patterns of Intimate Relationships.* New York: Quill, 1997.

Lerner, Sharon. "Good and Bad Marriage, Boon and Bane to Health." *New York Times.* October 22, 2002, p. F5.

Lindbergh, Anne Morrow. *Gift from the Sea.* reissue ed. New York: Pantheon, 1991.

Mead, Margaret. *Male and Female.* New York: William Morrow, 1949.

Morgan, Robin. *Saturday's Child: A Memoir.* New York: W. W. Norton, 2001.

Northrup, Christiane. *The Wisdom of Menopause: Creating Physical and Emotional Health and Healing During the Change.* New York: Bantam, 2001.

Orman, Suze. *The 9 Steps to Financial Freedom.* New York: Three Rivers Press, 2000.

Pagels, Elaine. *The Gnostic Gospels.* New York: Vintage Books, 1989.

Pederson, Rena with Dr. Lee Smith. *What's Next? Women Redefining Their Dreams in the Prime of Life.* New York: Perigee Books, 2001.

Perls, Frederick S. *Gestalt Therapy Verbatim,* revised ed. Highland, NY: Gestalt Journal Press, 1992.

Pinker, Steven. *The Blank Slate: The Modern Denial of Human Nature.* New York: Viking, 2002.

Pogrebin, Letty Cottin. *Getting Over Getting Older: An Intimate Journey.* Boston: Little, Brown and Company, 1996.

Rechtschaffen, Stephan. *Timeshifting: Creating More Time to Enjoy Your Life.* New York: Doubleday, 1996.

Restak, Richard. *The Secret Life of the Brain.* Washington D.C.: Joseph Henry Press, 2001.

Rossellini, Isabella. *Some of Me.* New York: Random House, 1997.

Rubenfeld, Ilana. *The Listening Hand: Self-Healing Through the Rubenfeld Synergy Method of Talk and Touch.* New York: Bantam Books, 2000.

Schor, Juliet B. *The Overworked American: The Unexpected Decline of Leisure.* New York: Basic Books, 1992.

Schwartz, Pepper. *Love Between Equals: How Peer Marriage Really Works.* New York: The Free Press, 1994.

Seaman, Barbara. *The Greatest Experiment Ever Performed on Women: Exploding the Estrogen Myth.* New York: Hyperion, 2003.

———. *The Doctors' Case Against the Pill.* Alameda, CA: Hunter House, Inc., 1995.

Sedlar, Jeri and Rick Miners. *Don't Retire, Rewire! 5 Steps to Fulfilling Work That Fuels Your Passion, Suits Your Personality, or Fills Your Pocket.* New York: Alpha Books, 2003.

Sheehy, Gail. *New Passages: Mapping Your Life Across Time.* New York: Ballantine Books, 1995.

Sher, Barbara. *It's Only Too Late If You Don't Start Now: How to Create Your Second Life at Any Age.* New York: Dell Trade Paperback, 1998.

Smith, J. Walker and Ann Clurman. *Rocking the Ages: The Yankelovich Report on Generational Marketing.* New York: HarperBusiness, 1997.

Steinem, Gloria. *Revolution from Within: A Book of Self-Esteem.* Boston: Little, Brown and Company, 1992.

———. *Outrageous Acts and Everyday Rebellions.* New York: Henry Holt and Company, 1995.

Strauch, Barbara. *The Primal Teen: What the New Discoveries About the Teenage Brain Tell Us About Our Kids.* New York: Doubleday, 2003.

Tavris, Carol. *The Mismeasure of Woman: Why Women Are Not the Better Sex, the Inferior Sex, or the Opposite Sex.* New York: Touchstone, 1992.

Taylor, Shelley, E. Klein, C. Laura, B. P. Lewis, T. L. Gruenewald, R.A.R. Gurung, and J. A. Updegraff. "Biobehavioral Responses to Stress in Females: Tend-and-Befriend, Not Fight-or-Flight." *Psychological Review.* July 2000, pp. 411–29.

Trafford, Abigail. *My Time: Making the Most of the Rest of Your Life.* New York: Basic Books, 2003.

Tyler, Anne. *Back When We Were Grownups.* New York: Ballantine Books, 2001.

Vaillant, George E. *Aging Well: Surprising Guideposts to a Happier Life.* Boston: Little, Brown and Company, 2002.

Weitzman, Lenore J. *The Divorce Revolution: The Unexpected Social and Economic Consequences for Women and Children in America.* New York: Free Press, 1985.

Wolf, Naomi. *The Beauty Myth: How Images of Beauty Are Used Against Women.* New York: William Morrow and Company, 1991.

Woolf, Virginia. *Three Guineas.* San Diego, CA: Harcourt, 1938.

Zuboff, Shoshana and James Maxmin. *The Support Economy: Why Corporations Are Failing Individuals and the Next Episode of Capitalism.* New York: Viking, 2002.

Web Sites and Organizations

AARP
www.aarp.org
The leading organization in the United States for people aged fifty and older. Features news, resources, and publications including the *AARP Bulletin* and *AARP The Magazine.*

Age Beat
www.asaging.org/agebeat/
A free newsletter of the Journalists Exchange on Aging. Features news, updates from the American Society on Aging, and links.

The Bag Lady Prevention Plan
www.bagladyprevention.com
Strategies for retirement and other midlife dilemmas. An online community for women over fifty. Features a newsletter, articles, and forums.

The Carole Hyatt Leadership Forum
www.carolehyatt.com
A resource for women embarking on the process of changing careers, changing jobs, becoming entrepreneurs or reenergizing a career that has stalled. Offers the Carole Hyatt Leadership Forum "New Perspectives Workshop" followed by Women's E-groups meeting monthly.

Center for the Advancement of Women
www.advancewomen.org
Founded by Fay Wattleton, former president of Planned Parenthood, the group conducts surveys by women, for women, about women.

Center for Women's Business Research
www.nfwbo.org
Information about women business owners and their enterprises worldwide.

Civic Ventures
www.civicventures.org
A national nonprofit organization founded by Marc Freedman to expand the contributions of older Americans to society, and to help transform the aging of American society into a source of individual and social renewal. Features publications, projects, and resources.

Catalyst
www.catalystwomen.org
Catalyst is the premier nonprofit research and advisory organization working to advance women in business, with offices in New York, San Jose, and Toronto. The leading source of information on women in business for the past four decades, Catalyst has the knowledge and tools that help companies recruit, retain, and advance top talent and enable women to reach their potential. Web site features publications, research, news, and a membership option.

The Dana Foundation
www.dana.org
A site for brain information. The Dana Press features free publications, *Brain in the News* and *BrainWork*.

Dr. Northrup.com: Empowering Women's Wisdom
www.drnorthrup.com
Dr. Christiane Northup's Web site features women's health information and news, online journals, health quizzes, and a store.

Foundation for Women's Wellness
1000 South Race Street, Denver, CO 80209
An organization founded by Dr. Lila Nachtigall and her daughter Ellen Biben to support research in women's health. Publishes a newsletter.

International Longevity Center
www.ilcusa.org
A nonprofit, nonpartisan research, policy, and education organization whose mission is to help societies around the world address issues of population aging and longevity in positive and constructive ways, and to highlight older people's productivity and contributions to their families and to society as a whole.

Kaiser Family Foundation
www.kff.org
A nonprofit, private foundation focusing on the major health-care issues facing the nation. Features extensive studies and reports.

The Kinsey Institute
www.kinseyinstitute.org
Promotes interdisciplinary research and scholarship in the fields of human sexuality, gender, and reproduction. Features publications, library, research programs, and resources.

Lauren Hutton's Good Stuff
www.laurenhutton.com
An online store with Lauren Hutton's makeup line—geared toward women, not girls.

Menopause Magic
www.menopausemagic.com
A New York–based site created by Dr. Patricia Yarberry Allen, obstetrician and gynecologist at the New York Hospital-Cornell Medical Center. The site is the link for the New York Menopause Center. Also has links to the New York Menopause Research Foundation, Menopause Mentors, and articles.

Mother's Grace
www.mothersgrace.com
Jyoti's Web site featuring her published works, upcoming projects, and more.

National Women's Health Network
www.nwhn.org
The National Women's Health Network develops and promotes a critical analysis of health issues in order to affect policy and support consumer decision making. The network aspires to a health-care system that is guided by social justice and reflects the needs of diverse women.

North American Menopause Society
www.menopause.org
The leading scientific nonprofit organization devoted to promoting women's health during midlife and beyond through an understanding of

menopause. This site contains information on perimenopause, early menopause, menopause symptoms, and long-term health effects of estrogen loss and a wide variety of therapies to enhance health.

Odyssey: School for the Second Half of Life
www.exed.hbs.edu/programs/ody/
An on-campus program at Harvard Business School led by professor Shoshana Zuboff.

Older Women's League
www.owl-national.org
The only national grassroots membership organization to focus solely on issues unique to women as they age, the Older Women's League (OWL) strives to improve the status and quality of life for midlife and older women. The site has health and retirement information, news, and links to local chapters.

Outward Bound
www.outwardboundwilderness.org
Outward Bound USA's official Web site. Look under "Special Focus Courses" for women-only programs and adult renewal programs. For programs in more than twenty countries. Visit Outward Bound International at www.outwardbound.net.

Red Hat Society
www.redhatsociety.com
The worldwide social phenomenon for celebrating women over fifty. Over twenty thousand chapters. Features news, links, and convention information.

Retirement or WHAT NEXT?
www.retirementorwhatnext.com
Transitions for women over fifty who want to make the most of life and wish to: redefine work, consider the possibilities, express creativity, and ponder what's next. Provides workshops, discussion groups, and individual consultations.

SeniorNet

www.seniornet.org

A nonprofit organization of computer-using adults, age fifty and older. SeniorNet's mission is to provide older adults education for and access to computer technologies to enhance their lives and enable them to share their knowledge and wisdom. The site features Web courses, a learning center, research papers and studies, news, and an online community forum where all individuals fifty and older, whether or not they are members of SeniorNet, are welcome to participate in online communities and hundreds of discussion topics.

Smith College Ada Comstock Scholars Program

www.smith.edu/admission/ada.php

Established in 1975, this program at Smith College enables women of nontraditional college age to complete a bachelor of arts degree at a realistic pace, either part time or full time. The program combines the rigorous academic challenges of Smith with flexibility for women beyond the traditional college age by providing options for reduced course loads, special academic advising, career counseling, and diverse housing options.

Suze Orman

www.suzeorman.com

Information about Suze Orman's books, television program, contact information, and other resources.

The Transition Network

www.thetransitionnetwork.org

Network that helps women move from the career and family stage of life to the next phase, with an emphasis on sharing professional and personal expertise among members. Features group volunteer projects, newsletter, resources. Currently based in the New York City area with plans to expand.

U.S. Census Bureau

www.census.gov

Resource for publications and reports from the Census Bureau with population, housing, economic, and geographic data.

Wellesley Centers for Women (WCW)
www.wcwonline.org
The nation's largest women's research center, WCW is the alliance of the Center for Research on Women and the Stone Center at Wellesley College. Features publications, news, analysis, and resources.

When Work Works
www.whenworkworks.org
A project undertaken in collaboration with the Families and Work Institute (www.familiesandwork.org) on workplace effectiveness and workplace flexibility. As part of the nationwide initiative, the Web site has resources and information for employers, managers, employees, and the public at large.

WomanSage
www.womansage.com
A nonprofit organization dedicated to empowering, educating, and fostering mentoring relationships among midlife women with a news-based Web site, a quarterly journal, annual conferences, monthly salons, and small special-interest groups. Based in Orange County, California, and currently in the process of chapter development nationwide. National memberships available.

Women's eNews
www.womensenews.com
An independent news agency that covers issues of particular concern to women and provides women's perspectives on public policy. Subscribe and receive daily news stories or summaries and/or a weekly summary. Subscriptions are free.

The Woodhull Institute
www.woodhull.org
Provides ethical leadership training and professional development for women.

Yankelovich
www.yankelovich.com
Yankelovich is a consultancy providing information, database, and custom marketing services. The site features information for businesses including the *Yankelovich Monitor*.

Index